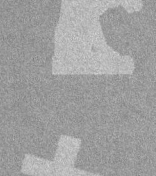

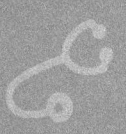

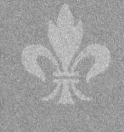

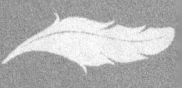

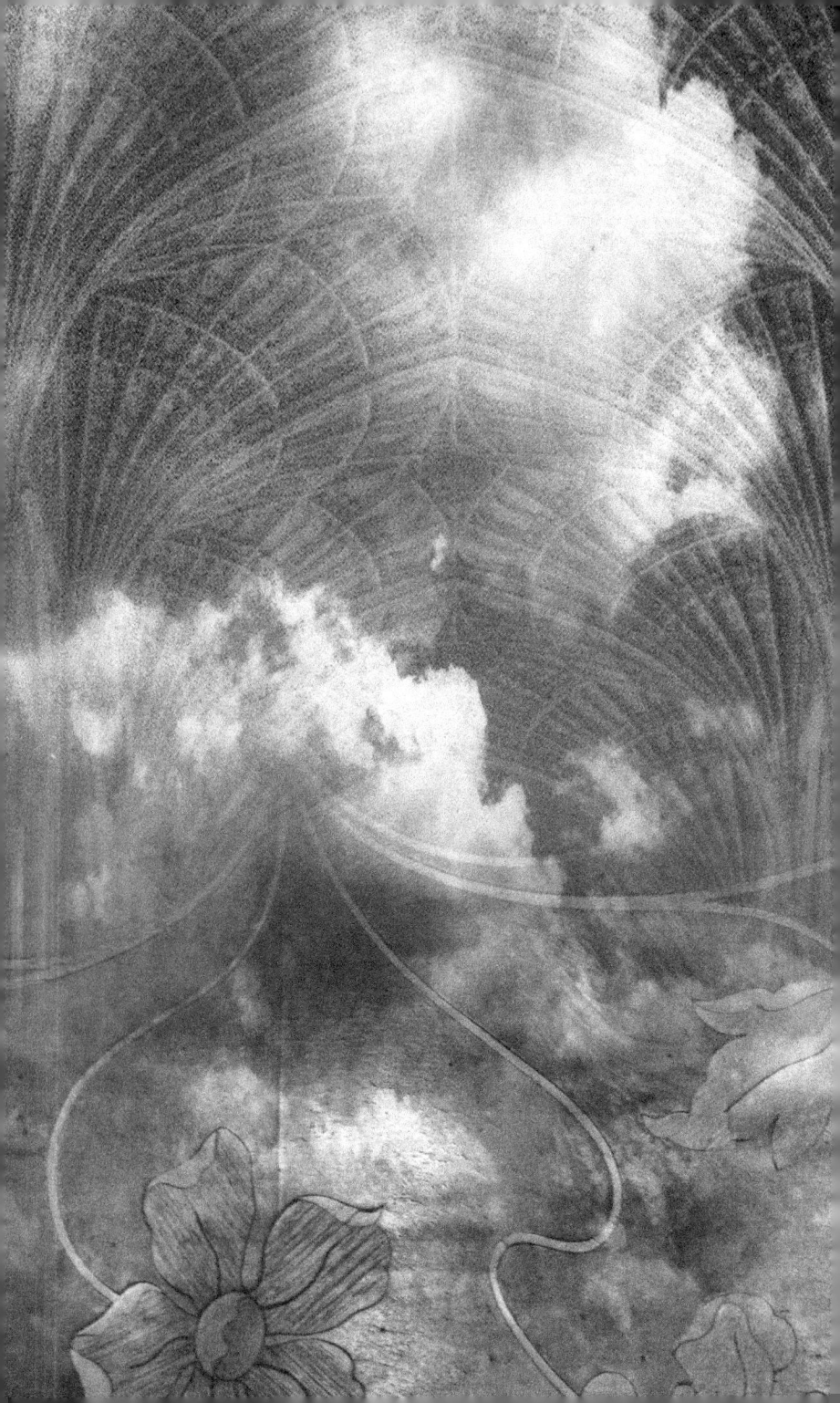

The Evolve Fertility Series
by Beth Alderman, MD, MPH

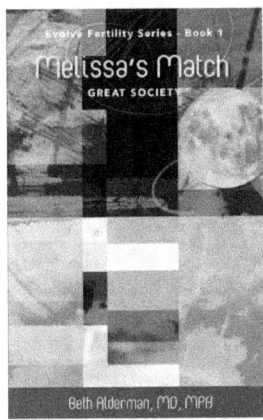

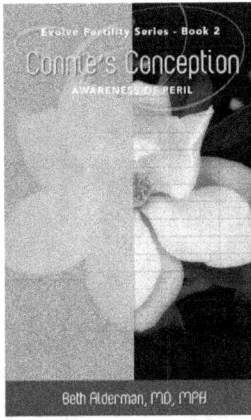

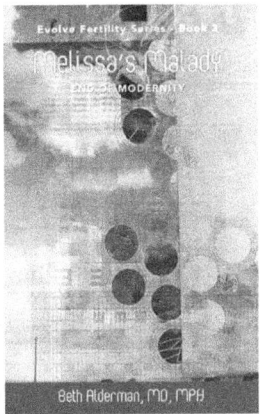

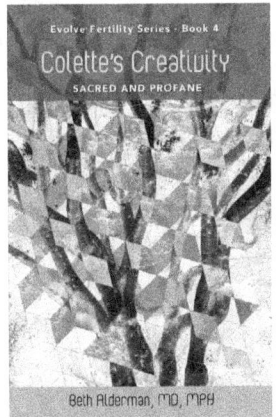

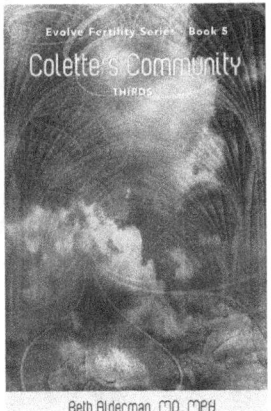

Colette's Community

THIRDS

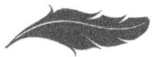

Book Five of the
Evolve Fertility Series

Beth Alderman, MD, MPH

LIVING FUTURE BOOKS · ASHLAND, OREGON

Colette's Community: Thirds
by Beth Alderman, MD, MPH

© 2019 Future Medicine, LLC
www.LivingFutureBooks.com

For related online courses visit
www.LivingFutureCourses.com

Editor: Julie Clayton
Cover Art: www.BruceBayard.com
Book Design: www.BookSavvyStudio.com

Library of Congress Control Number: 2019903852
ISBN: 978-1-7321110-4-2

First Edition
Printed in the United States of America

Contents

To Barbara and Kathy

Sex can lift our attention upward and offer a visionary experience of life based in love and passion that is the equal of any abstract philosophy or highly spiritual form of contemplation. Sex is not only earthy; it is also sublime.

—THOMAS MOORE in *The Soul of Sex*

The generative powers of the male that come at puberty are meant to solve the larger cosmic purpose of generation. They are not to serve the individual ego, or even the ego of the family or nation or tribe, but the overall purpose of nature itself... The Green Man [has] a rich sexuality that does not draw attention to itself but embodies the ongoing sexual and creative energy of the universe.

—MATTHEW FOX in *The Hidden Spirituality of Men*

1

The Yarra Valley

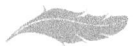

As I wait at the Lilydale train station and look for Reggie's car, I collect my thoughts. After living the slow life in the States for almost three months, I returned to St. Kilda last week to learn the local wine market from Lisa, who took me around to wine shops, wineries, and tastings to educate my palate. Then, yesterday, she took me to get a makeover that Reggie had arranged for me at her favorite shops on Acland Street, which prepared me to present Yarra Spur wines as fashion-forward and cutting-edge. Lisa's working persona is exacting and ambitious and opinionated; I can see why Andy is a little afraid of her. She brought out my obedience and lingering perfectionism and did nothing to put me at ease in my new vixen's clothing. I have yet to strike the right stance for my new role in wine sales.

But right now I'm more worried about Reg. When we spoke on the phone last night, she was her usual bright self but for a note of tension in her voice. Given her usual poise, even the smallest sign of distress is worrisome. I don't think she and Andy have been overworking, or straining to adapt to their new jobs. The work is well within their capabilities. I think it's because we left Denton Stables the morning after the debacle of the tent and they dove straight into work, leaving her no time to grieve. Andy and Lisa are both a bit concerned, and Lisa charged me with looking after Reg and making her life easier.

I decide to tell her only the funny stories from my trip and to edit out the rest. I do my best to emulate Reg's usual state—as best I can recall it after these months away—and then run my mind back over the highlights: my time in Colorado with Melissa where we were snowed in by an unexpected blizzard; a lively and only a little decadent Thanksgiving in New Orleans with my brother; and an arctic Christmas in Illinois with Maman, where we were joined by Sean and all the relatives who lived within two hundred miles. They helped me to fully reconcile with Maman. I don't know what my true-blue brother said to her, but it melted her heart.

I will not tell Reg that I only thought of Steve when someone else insisted; that there is a blank where he and his family were, about which I feel only relief rather than the loss of twenty years. I will not tell her that Sean is drinking too much and is restive in family life and so is philandering as our father did, which knowledge has created a wound in my heart where the men I loved so blindly used to be. I am struggling to love those who defined my ideas of husbanding and fathering, and paradoxically am yearning for a man of my own whom I will know and love through and through, and who will never disappoint me because I will expect nothing, and will allow every happy accident or intention to be a joyous surprise.

I will not tell Reg how difficult it is for me to recognize and take to heart my childhood friend Melissa, who is sick and whose family scorns her. She seems desperate and yet does nothing to help herself, everything to help her family. It drives me mad with frustration. And still she disdains any non-Jewish spirituality and practices that could ease her pain. Surely it is natural to want to feel better?

I am lost in thought so long that I don't see Reg until she stops her car in front of me and hops out to open its boot—its trunk. I rush toward her and she gives me a hug. It is like the hug she gave me last year at this time, when she met me at the Melbourne airport and squeezed away the tense chill that had become the deepest habit of my life. As I return her warmth, I say, "I can't tell you how much I missed you and how glad I am to be back!"

Reg pulls back and looks me in the eye. "We didn't scare you away?"

"No, no. I've come home—for the while at least."

Reggie releases a telltale sigh of tension. She stows my bag, we hop in, and we're off. I share my censored story, which amuses her. We are soon in exotic-to-me but lovely country, some of which looks wild. When she turns up a drive, and passes several bikes and is slowed by several cars ahead of us, I am amazed at the winery's popularity. It is beautiful, with expansive lawns, lush vineyards, and an old Edwardian farmhouse of white-painted brick that is now the tasting room. Reg continues on past the visitor parking to the gravel employee parking lot. There she jumps out and I follow like a crazed fan of wine, barely able to contain the excitement of moving on with this new life.

"Our vineyard is one of the smaller ones," Reggie says, smiling and drawing in a gulping breath as if drinking the air. The bright sun fades her freckles and hennaed hair and turns her denim eyes icy blue. "We don't have a restaurant with a view, just this tasting room, but the Age featured us as part of a school holiday excursion in spite of that. It's been great for sales, but mad, absolutely mad, every day all day."

Reggie glances at her watch and strides away between two rows of parked cars. Beads of sweat trickle from her hairline, and her shirt and shorts cling to her back. A fine gray dust rises from the gravel and clings to her scuffed shoe boots. I grab my bag, shake out the gauzy folds of my new peach-colored dress, and follow, stepping hurriedly but gingerly in my new stilettos. We pass couples lounging on wrought-iron lace benches in the rose garden; families picnicking in the shade of gum trees brightened by showy birds; an elderly man in a wrinkled white suit emerging from the rear door of the white house, his face transformed by fun.

"I can stay today," Reggie calls over her shoulder, "but you'll be on your own after."

Behind us rise new outbuildings of corrugated metal and wood that stand out, bright and angular, against undulant fields of wide-set vines. Beyond, the forest of the great divide with its tufted, gray-green gums recedes into a blurry, distant blanket. Soon the formal rose garden that stretches for ten meters to the wrap-around veranda of the farmhouse is also behind us, and Reg is ducking in a side door. She pauses inside a small office to smile and say cheerily, "The important thing—and I know you'll be spot-on with that—is to be gracious."

"What if they have questions?"

"Answer if you can, give out leaflets if you can't, and come get Andy or me if you must."

Reggie dives through the facing door beyond the workstation and into the cool, damp air of the low-lit tasting room. The interior reminds me of an oversized crate that smells of wine-soaked corks and rotting wood. Its still, damp air echoes with the scraping of boxes, the clinking of wine bottles, and ripples of low conversation punctuated by sips and spits. As my eyes adjust, I see bottles everywhere: standing on tables, lying in gift boxes, resting on racks, and waiting in stacked wooden crates. The narrow aisles between displays of bottles are thronged with crowds of shoppers, some kneeling or stooping, some stretching to read labels.

"You're bloody late!" booms a voice from the far side of the room. It came from a walrus-like man in a bush hat and moustache who is standing behind a marble-topped counter with his thick arms folded over his belly. He has fixed his tiny, close-set eyes on Reggie.

Reggie darts across the room and returns cheerfully, "Mr. Wheeler, I'd like you to meet my friend from the States, Colette Connolly." She sweeps her arm in my direction and says, "Colette, this is Mr. Oliver Wheeler, the owner of Yarra Spur."

I extend my hand as I pull up my posture and try to put on a suitable persona. My mind flits like a dragonfly—from Maine farming women, to city babes, to society ladies—and lands in the safety of my childhood role of nun in disguise.

Mr. Wheeler ignores my hand and my posture and my persona. He inspects me suspiciously and mutters, "Bloody kiwi." He is presumably insulting my predecessor, a student from New Zealand who was called away on a family emergency. Mr. Wheeler lumbers out from behind the counter. He is wearing short shorts and shoe boots that seem comical to me, but that in Aussie eyes invoke a working-class street tough. "I hope you're not as lazy as that last Yank. Bloody Septics."

He is the first fair dinkum bloke of his generation that I have met, which may be the reason that he enters my perceptions as a stereotype. His epithets date him. Aussies can no longer mock Americans by comparing our country to a septic tank; they too have welcomed "the poor, tired, and huddled masses" of the world since the end of WWII, and many recall with heart the American forces that opposed the Japanese invaders who threatened the north.

Reggie turns to two lanky men idling at the counter and shakes their hands with a glowing smile. "I'm Reggie Pappas, managing oenologist. Have you tried the Botrytis? We had great reviews of our other wines, but the critics missed this one, and it's gorgeous."

The men look at me. They stare at me as if my breasts are headlights that freeze them in place. Men have been responding to me oddly since the sexy makeover, which includes the peach-colored folly of a dress that is overexposing my pushed-up breasts and narrowing my waist with a corset.

I follow Reg around the counter and watch her take two glasses from a shelf. She uncorks a bottle of amber-colored wine and pours out two one-ounce samples. She hands me the bottle as if to indicate that I should pour more on request. "I'll leave you to it, then."

One of the men, a handsome redhead with angular features, fixes his eyes on my cleavage. I nearly lose my nerve, but have worked retail before, and instinctively turn my tension into a sale. I envelop his shy, bent-nosed mate in a velvety blanket of sensual solicitude. The first man's face flickers in irritation. The other warms to me. Both end up buying gift boxes.

The first hour passes in a halting dance of false steps and near collisions. By closing time, I can adroitly twist my wrist to avoid drawing arcs of red drops on the counter and readily answer common questions. Even so, the job feels surprisingly difficult. I am enchanted by the gregarious antipodean manners, and can tune in to the accent, but my instincts are off. If I emulate Daphne, my favorite waitress at the Koffee Klatsch in Maine, who neither hurries nor neglects her customers, I feel like a doting nanny. If I try to emulate Reggie, I realize that there is no trick to what she does. It's what she is that I admire, and that draws everyone toward her as to the sun.

Usually thinking of the past is like looking back on a long sleep, or the time before I was born, but selling wine reminds me of summers when I worked for businesses down the coast, like the cycling shop, the dog groomer's, or the accountant's office. I enjoyed the challenge of becoming indispensable to harried or ornery business owners who disliked the public. I was the most gracious of my fellow workers, but I have never possessed Reggie's easy grace. She is kind to confused neophytes, and delightful with jaded wine snobs. She can talk about value with investors, and the slow savoring of flavors with gourmands. She knows her business, and even when hauling crates in the field she embodies class. Nothing fazes or sticks to her, not broken bottles, petulant employees, whining children, cranky critics, or starry-eyed admirers who presume to intimacy.

"Great crowd, wasn't it?" she says as my first working day draws to a close. "Everyone keen for a bit of fun. No one tired and emotional."

"Do you think so? I'm tipsy just from the smell."

Reggie laughs. "Better hold your nose, then. I need you clear-headed when you close out the till."

When only three visitors remain, she takes me through the room like an agent going over nicks and quirks on a rent-a-wreck. I start the shiny new dishwasher, put clean glasses in rough-hewn cupboards, and stack linens in a sideboard by the big dining table in the library, where Reggie holds classes and other events. I immediately forget some items and their purposes, but others stay with me, like the Irish linens that the owner's wife, Marilyn, keeps for family gatherings. Each piece has quirks too, like the cupboard you can open only if you lift the door handle up and to the right.

As I empty the dishwasher, the office door opens with a bang and Mr. Wheeler trumpets harshly, "I'll show you around now."

Reggie tips her head to cue me to follow.

Mr. Wheeler launches on a circuit of the floor, pointing and proclaiming opinions like a member of the Australian Parliament insulting the opposition. In a far corner he points to a stack of crates. "They grow better wood up in Taggerty, but the bloody idiots use foreign pinewood. If a crate breaks you'll clean it up and pay the damages. If you can't handle it, get help. You Yanks want to sue every time you stuff up your backs."

"I'm pretty strong."

Mr. Wheeler trudges grimly out of the back door into the heat. Ignoring the visitors on the back veranda, he shuffles across the gravel lot and into the lukewarm stillness of the nearest corrugated metal outbuilding. Leading the way down the middle of the plant's floor, he dismisses Reggie's glass-walled laboratory with a wave, points out a bottling apparatus perfunctorily, and curses American consumers for liking cork stoppers instead of screw tops.

After exiting onto a patch of lawn, though, his tone changes. He points to the trellises at the far end of the adjacent field and says confidentially, "I planted my last vines twenty years ago, but there were vines here a hundred and fifty years before. The depression of 1890 shut down some of the wineries in my great grandfather's time. But we're fair battlers here at the Spur, so we expanded to include the old McDairmuid vines planted by Reggie's ancestors."

When he enters the far building, he slows and softens. Before exiting the pungent air of the barrel room, he stops to pat a barrel and declares, "American oak. Wouldn't use anything else." Back in the tasting room, he finishes *sotto voce*, "Don't mind the bloody pounces and tall poppies come in here. Reggie coddles 'em, but I say the poms down the road can have the whole bloody lot."

"Thank you for the tour, Mr. Wheeler."

"You'll do all right, then." He gives a slight nod and plods outside.

I return to the tasting room and follow the sounds of clinking bottles to the far aisle. "He's the brashest bloke I've seen so far!"

Reggie straightens the last stack of crates. "He certainly took to you! I've never seen him like that."

"Really?" I laugh.

"Ah, yeah. He can be pretty harsh, especially to new staff."

"Where's his wife?"

"We used to see her a lot, but she's moved up to Lilydale to care for her sick mother." Reggie shelves a misplaced bottle and nods her approval. "Ready for tea?"

"Famished. But where's home?"

She gestures vaguely in the direction of the front stairs. "When they fixed up the tasting room they converted the upstairs into a suite. I made a deal to live in it for a while in lieu of a signing bonus."

"Great. How do we close up?"

Reggie shows me how to reconcile the electronic till, which requires a fresh ink cartridge and new roll of paper for receipts and reports.

I retrieve my bag and drag it up to Reggie's room. In her delightful loft, which takes up the whole of the upper floor, I immediately feel at home. She has done it up beautifully. Under the western eaves on the left, milky curtains caress a breeze before pooling on the floor. Inside the curtains, the bright lights of a kitchenette reflect off the wooden dining table that, judging from the pile of papers and books, doubles as her desk. Under the eastern eaves to the right, a king-sized bed mounded with pillows stands in front of the opening of a wide alcove. Between the alcove and kitchenette are doors that open to a toilet and bathroom. In the center of the room a large sofa bed stands open, outfitted with an inviting set of blue and yellow Provençale linens. On either side sit antique end tables and overstuffed armchairs.

I am delighted and impressed. "Pretty fancy digs you got here."

"Don't let Wheeler hear you say that! He'll want to charge me."

I drop my bag beside the sofa bed and take a seat on a creaky dining chair to pull off my new shoes and look at the red imprints they left on my skin. "The best thing about fancy new shoes is taking them off."

Reggie takes a stack of pre-made crêpes from her freezer. "Collo, why don't you pour us a little cider while I bung a few crêpes on the burner?"

"Sure thing." I search her small refrigerator and cabinets until I find what I need to pour out two clay cups of French cider. "I didn't realize the sacrifice you had made when you took the job with Wheeler."

"Ah, look, Wheeler is a brilliant farmer with prime land. He can grow gorgeous grapes when others are stuck with bald spurs. And he's willing to let me develop in all sides of the business." She pokes her head in the fridge and then takes out a head of butter lettuce. "I've tried to help him with his foul state of mind, but he clings to it like a barnacle."

I rummage for the rest of the fixings, finding a wooden salad bowl and filling it with a lettuce and shredded savoy cabbage, and dressing it with olive oil and a balsamic vinaigrette with shredded parmesan from her sparsely-filled fridge.

"You seem to be moving in double time," I say, remembering Lisa's request. "I could make dinner for both of us from now on."

"Ah, that'd be great. I'm busier than I'd like right now. I don't see Graeme often and when I do he gives me energy—but he's tiring of it."

"Do you want to sit tonight?"

Reggie sighs in relief. "A daily meditation practice would be a real pick-me-up."

"How about once tonight and then daily in the early morning?"

"It'd have to be really early, 4:30 or 5:00."

"No problem—as long as I don't have to take care of any chickens first."

"I did get a few chooks."

"Really? I'll take care of them after," I laugh.

Reggie serves out two crêpes. I put a baguette and lump of foil-wrapped butter on the table. We sit down to eat. My fatigue disappears when my taste buds encounter the delightful musk of aged Gruyère, the tang of well-aged ham, and the crisp edge of a perfectly browned crêpe. "Reggie, this crêpe is as good as Maman's, and that's saying a lot."

Reggie sips her cider and leans back, her shoulders slumping slightly. After a minute, the glow behind her eyes rekindles. "Ah, it's great to eat at home and not have to drink wine!"

"Don't you usually eat at home?"

"No, no. When I don't have to look after guests I have to dine at another winery, or in town. It's part of the job. Wine is meant to enhance the taste of food, so the business of fine wine is all about fine dining. In fact, I have a few dishes I'd like you to make for the tasting classes we offer in fall and winter."

"I'd like that."

"Thanks for coming back early. The tasting room is key to our viability. No sales, no viticulture or viniculture."

"I'm happy to do it, and happy to be back. I have at least three months on my tourist visa."

"Gyogos thinks his lawyer may be able to get you a work visa as an artist or French cooking teacher."

"Thanks for looking into that. I do want to pull my weight, and I presume the tasting room work will trail off after the holidays."

Reggie nods. "We'll probably go to weekends-only in March, and may close for the winter this year."

"Do you have other work for me?"

"I do have a project in mind," Reggie says hesitantly. "We have some old cottages here that could be renovated for a bed and breakfast, or for seasonal weekend retreats. It would be good for business, and with your cooking and art and Andy's help with the heavy work, you could create an income stream to support your salary."

"What's your timeframe and budget?"

"Don't have any yet, but the budget would probably be small. Retro décor and lots of paint—including art—would do a lot to offset that disadvantage."

"I see murals in my future. Should be fun."

"Ah, it's a relief to hear you say that."

"Why don't you go have a soak in the bath? I'll clean up here and you can save the water for me."

Later, when I am fresh and have reveled in the soft bed, I am tired and yet exhilarated. I savor the process of falling asleep by dwelling on today's wonders. The soft fog of the early morning resolving into hazy mist, and then into clouds that drifted east to settle on the hillside. Gentle breezes stroking the brown earth, riffling the high summer leaves, and brushing clouds gently over the divide.

Once again I see the last light of day touch the trellises entwined with grape vines shaded by parasol leaves and dotted with pendant clusters of ripening grapes, the gray-green gumtree forest scrimshawed by sinuous branches and tufted treetops; the snaking road to Taggerty that parts the forest and outlines crumbling rows of cliffs and the black stony tusk from which the winery takes its name. It is easy to fall in love with country Victoria, where culture and civilization coexist with the wild. It becomes the stuff of my dreams.

As I am dozing off, the night's murmurs are interrupted by a coughing sound that sends my body into a state of alarm. I open my eyes and listen. I hear it again. "What was that?"

"What? The owl?"

"No, not an owl. It isn't hooting, it's coughing."

"It's barking. The owl's a barking owl. It's nested in the red gum."

"Really? No! Next you're going to be telling me about the Cheshire cat."

"You mean the Tazzie tiger?"

"What? No! I mean the smiling cat from Alice in Wonderland."

"Feel like you've tumbled down a rabbit hole, do you?"

"No! Back in community with you and Andy I feel like I'm in a wonder-filled land!"

2

Harvest

alk, cradle, snip, nestle. Walk, cradle, snip, nestle. The mantra of harvest is motion, a line dance with drying vine leaves that have spent themselves for the sake of juice-filled fruit. It is a loving meditation on the abundance of an earth that we enrich with joy and gratitude. Now, while my body is fresh, I am delighted to leave the physical stagnation of sales and to satisfy my body's desire for purposeful patterns of movement. My mind is free to explore the body and its wisdom as Reg and I had been discussing over dinner each day before the harvest swept us all out of our daily routines.

Reg and I had focused on being and becoming and ignored doing—except with regard to sexuality, a topic that I do my best to ignore. Early in life, my body was patterned by play, dance, housework, school, and industrial work. I was most often disciplined by a clock or machine until the farm brought me closer to nature and nurture. Now many patterns are converging that I once thought modern but now recognize as primal—as shapers of human evolution.

An hour into the day, though, my shoulders ache and my mind grows numb. The harvest ritual begins to remind me of the dance of the dead that served an assembly line in a factory. The line's vast array of great mechanisms excited and terrorized me with their pounding and grinding and disregard for human life. We could only wear our helmets, remain alert, and hope. But while the repetition here feels similar, everything else is new. I work hard, but am willing and free, and the end is in sight. I hone my rhythm so that my yield is resilient to the pauses created as I wipe my hairline with my sleeve, dodge a clod of dirt, or roll my shoulders to loosen and refresh their muscles. The wisdom I learned from engineers allows me to move quickly down the row, faster than men too young to attend to time and too strong to gauge their efforts.

My mind is still free to wander back to yesterday, when Reggie tasted the grapes and analyzed them for sugar and acid. She watched the horizon for clues as to the weather, and consulted the official weather reports. Though she would have liked to let the grapes ripen for another week at least, she decided that the risk of rain was too great, and that it was time to harvest. Andy called in the friends and family members who come out every harvest to help with picking and told them to meet in the north field at sunrise. Ruth and Melanie and their children came out, as they often do now to see Lisa's baby, whom they still call sprout because Lisa and Andy cannot agree on a name for her.

Because the number of customers has declined steadily since the school holidays, I had time to help, and so was pleasantly surprised when Reggie asked me over dinner, "Want to try your hand at picking? It's tough yakka, but it's hours and dollars to the good."

Step, cradle, snip, nestle, step, and shift. Step cradle, snip, nestle, step, and shift. At sunrise, Oliver's great hands turned surprisingly gentle when he showed us how to caress the delicate clusters of fruit, and to cut them deftly from the vine and nestle them in upturned crates. The air was cool then, and the pale sun slowly revealed the canes and shoulder-high trellis wires that hold the branches that hold the fruit and leaves. The growing light outlined both gross and fine details of the perfectly pruned arches of mature beryl leaves, and the clusters of jade and garnet grapes.

Step, cradle, snip, nestle, step, and shift. I long to talk and joke with Carolyn, the sturdy grandmother with short gray hair and quick smile who came with me to the south field to pick the cabernet grapes, but she is beginning to tire, and snapped at Andy for calling her Caro. When it is time to take our lunch break, we sit in silence and eat our sandwiches in the paltry shade of an arbor. We stare at the foliage and at the baby blue sky, which conceals the stars of the Southern Crux from our light-befuddled eyes.

I realize as food revives us that I can use a spiritual practice—*tonglen*—to turn the aches and pains that are overtaking my body into a purification practice that will strengthen my heart centers and leave me better able to shift my resting state of being toward love and joy.

Step, cradle, snip, nestle, step, and shift. Now, as I clip off the ripe fruit with my sharp knife, I breathe in my present pain and the errors of the past. I turn their destructive power on my harmful habits of mind, especially my unthinking obedience. I breathe in pain, and breathe out joy and peace. For a while, I keep up.

My thoughts return now to the flight from the States and my first week in St. Kilda, when my body's clock had yet to join me here, and I felt disoriented and displaced; and then to my first day at Yarra Spur winery, when a cyclone of alterations, new experiences, and intense exchanges re-patterned my body and planted in it the seeds of an entirely new life. I try to see what's next as I do every night when I go to the rose garden at dusk to gaze toward the horizon and ponder our ultimate destination.

Step, cradle, snip, nestle, step, and shift. As my pain increases, memory takes me back to the likewise painful thoughts of the farmhouse in Maine. My husband and in-laws are sitting together at the dining table discussing the next year's work, and the problem of making use of me. I escape into knitting. I knit twelve; crossover; knit twelve; purl thirty. I fill my mind with pattern, and with the beauty of wool provided by generous, unstinting nature through her fruitful sheep. I alter the practice to breathe in the pain of all of the pickers, which turns this evanescent trial into a ready habit of turning suffering into strength.

Step, cradle, snip, nestle, step, and shift. Hours on, my mind has sunk. I think of nothing but reaching the end of a row, where I can shift the sling of my crate to the opposite shoulder and drink deeply of sweet water. I am determined to do my part. I do what I can to overlook the pain in my shoulders and the creeping weakness in my hands. I move in to cool my ankles in the light breeze that filters through the widely set canes. *It's only pain*, I tell myself.

Step, cradle, snip, nestle, step, and shift. Gradually the yellow of the sun deepens, burnishing the vine leaves. I try to imagine Carolyn's face radiating joy, and to trust that I will someday become strong enough to share abundant joy with all who are in pain. But I am too tired to think of anything but motion. When the sun is five degrees above the horizon, I think only of making it to sunset, and to the respite of a quiet supper and early sleep. *Tomorrow's work is a problem for tomorrow.*

Suddenly I hear voices, and a tone of trouble. Andy is striding up the row. "Change in plans for tomorrow," he says grimly. "Evelyn got the call from Marilyn today. Her mother died this morning."

Carolyn puts her hand to her mouth. She is first cousin to Oliver's wife Marilyn and a neighbor of Evelyn, the wizened sack of bones who is Oliver's uncle and is handling the office and tasting room today.

"Better stop for the day, Carolyn. Marilyn wants your help with the wake. If you hurry you can get a ride to town with Evelyn and Oliver. Colette, tomorrow you'll pick until eleven and then handle the tasting room."

"Sure thing."

"And Reg says that she'll be running the Burnt Tree de-stemmer until late and not to wait for her."

"Okay."

Andy puts his hand on Carolyn's shaking shoulder and says kindly, "I'm sorry for your loss."

The next thing I know, it is morning, still before sunrise, and Reggie's alarm is sounding. She gets up with difficulty and grabs a day-old baguette. She comes with me to the fields to assess the progress of the harvest, and to invite everyone to the evening's wake. Our mood is heavy with the remembrance of death and the threat of rain. If we do not hurry, the rain will come and the grapes will fill with water, and so dilute their sugar and compromise the wine. I pick as fast and as long as I can and then rush up to shower and change just in time to open the tasting room at eleven.

There are no customers. I stand idly behind the counter feeling like a doll in a diorama. I know that I couldn't have kept up the pace of picking and am glad to have this respite, yet have the feeling that I am doing less than I could for Reggie and the rest. I recognize that this regret is laced with ambition as well as guilt, so I take a cloth from under the sink, dust the bottles in the aisles, and take pleasure in remembering that the beauties of the vineyard rely on the work that each of us is doing. I regret that the winery will soon open only by appointment, and that Andy will take on the task of receiving customers while I work on the cottages that I now realize will be a long shot because of the rapidly advancing development of weekend packages in the valley.

The phone rings, and I rush to answer. "Yarra Spur winery, Colette speaking. How may I help you today?

An engaging but unfamiliar male voice asks, "Colette? Colette Connelly?"

"Speaking."

"Melissa said I should call you."

I notice that his accent is American. "Sorry to be blunt, but who are you?"

"I'm Randall, a college friend of Melissa's. I'm in Sydney, just finishing up a few months' sabbatical. She suggested that I contact you before I leave."

"Oh! I'm happy to hear from any friend of Melissa." My mind races to place him. "Wait, weren't you her boyfriend at one time?"

"We were lovers in college, and got back in touch a few years ago. I've been wanting to see more of the country, and I have business in Melbourne, so I thought I might stop in to visit you on my way back to the States." He adds ingratiatingly, "That is, if you don't mind a visit from a total stranger who's a huge fan of your exquisite wines."

I leapt to the conclusion that Melissa suggested it. Then, an image of Grandma appears in my mind's eye. She is speaking of her desire to bring in guests from abroad. I see a snapshot of an ad in which Randall tells his well-connected American friends about Reggie's wines, and the wonderful weekend getaways that I could develop and host at the Spur. I decide that he could be the trial guest for a new wine country excursion that will create a job for me here.

"If you like, you could come out to Yarra Spur and stay in one of the old guest cottages on the property. I'm just redoing them in preparation for starting wine and cuisine weekend getaways."

"Fabulous! I'd love to see Melbourne, too." He says it the American way, as Mel Born. "Do you know the city?"

"I stayed there when I first came out, and I've been back a few times. I could meet your train or flight, and we could see some of the city before coming out to the Yarra. How does that sound?"

"Perfect! I have one more thing to ask, if it isn't too much."

"That depends. What is it?"

"My locum ends on March thirty-first so I'll be there for Pesach. I'd like to attend a seder."

"Pesach?"

"The feast of the Jewish holiday of Passover. You've heard of it?"

"I've heard of Passover."

"Don't worry about it. I can find a seder."

"Are you sure? My boss's friend Hal is probably hosting one."

"Melbourne has a strong Jewish community. I'm sure I could find one." I sense that he is trying to be polite.

"Let me ask my boss. She's very well connected."

"If it isn't too much trouble."

"Not at all. My pleasure."

"Great. I'll be in touch."

As I ring off, several customers come in. In quick succession I serve black-clad newlyweds from St. Kilda, a widower comforting himself with a new wine collection, and a busload of depressed Canadians from Regina, some of who are disappointed to find that we have no beer. Groups small and large pass through until the room hums with comings and goings, and the till is filled with income that I will be glad to report to Reggie and the others.

When the door whooshes closed with a deep sigh, I lock it and make a last circuit of the tasting room. In the far corner, past the last row of shelves, a couple is conversing quietly in Japanese, each fully absorbed in the other. I feel the ineffable interplay of yin and yang shimmering between them, their exploration of unborn possibility, and the tingling anticipation that a third entity could be coming into being through their intangible union. I wonder if it will be a spirit or brain child, a shared purpose or task, a family or community, or a mutual transformation that expands and spreads. I wonder that celibacy and meditation have attuned me to the generative energies of others. I greet them, tell them that we are closing, reopen the till with easy delight and send them on their way with an Irish blessing.

Later, I crunch up the gravel path, heels scuffing rhythmically past the darkening garden. I draw in the cooling air that smells of roses, and delight in the lingering lavender color that sunset painted on the sky and earth. Creeping loneliness has been dulling my senses and obscuring an intangible but undeniable ache. It hits me like a stinging slap: I am ready for a life bond, for those fruits of union that are usually obscured by bottled-up desire.

I see Reggie's silhouette rising from the parking lot next to her truck, which is evidently back from the de-stemmer. The timed floodlight snaps on. Reggie is speaking to Carolyn, who is leaning against the truck looking weary and low. "We'll follow you, then, shall we?"

"Yuh', yuh'," Carolyn replies, sighing deeply and climbing into a small car in which several pickers are waiting. The car rips out of the lot toward the highway, overdriving its headlights.

"Crikey!" Reggie stretches her arms and collapses into her car.

I join her in the car and ask, "So, how did it go today?"

"Burnt Tree's making trouble over the de-stemmer. I reckon

I'll be forced to leave the stems in the low-end wines this year." Reggie squeezes her eyelids together. "Ah, look, it's just the usual for harvest time. We'll keep at it, and we'll keep up."

I have never seen her so frustrated. She is spent. I say, "A good meal and a break might help, even if it is a wake."

"Andy says Wheeler's been drinking hard. Let's hope he doesn't make life worse for Marilyn. She's had some rough times with her mum. That's tough yakka, that is, caring for the dying. Harder than harvest work." As Reggie spins the car and speeds up the drive, she asks tensely, "I hope you sold some cases. Andy said it was slow."

"There was a rush at the end. We sold more today than all of last week."

Reggie grunts and relaxes her shoulders. "Thanks for that."

We speed along the highway. Just before Lilydale, Reggie makes a right on a curb-less street that runs through a spread-out suburb of brightly lit houses. Half a mile in, Reggie parks behind a string of cars and climbs out. I join her to cross the uneven street, shuffle across several wide grassy yards strewn with fallen paperbark, and climb the creaky front stairs of a frame house that stands open to the night. When we step inside, we see Oliver standing to our right in the front corner beside a stooped woman with raven-dyed hair and fine features. Her nose is red and chapped, and her eyes are set deeply into red-pink skin that looks like crumpled tissue paper. It must be Marilyn, whose expression reveals her loss.

The scene inside is not what I expected. The house is filled with people, but they are not showing the emotion that I expect from the Irish diaspora, or from Australians. Perhaps some are enervated by the work of the harvest, and others are unused to sending the deceased into the other world by expressing their accumulated love and loathing. They give the room the feel of a limbo where un-mourned souls might wait until the end of time.

The line of mourners snakes in from a side room into the living room, passing Oliver and Marilyn and then a buffet table laden with heavy potluck dishes. As we make our way to the end of the line, we nod to friends and family members. When we reach the adjacent room, we find our place by the deceased woman's body. It is laid out on a heavy antique table, head raised by a linen-clad pillow and body hidden by a starched, pressed sheet bordered by antique lace. A wizened white hand rests on her heart, holding a jade rosary. Her fine features echo those of her daughter. Above this solemn scene hangs a copy of a page from the Book of Kells framed in gilded wood.

Here, at least, a handful of drunken elders spin stories that will outlive her. A beer-swilling fat man recounts a ribald story about Marilyn's mother, while a pinched-faced thin woman contradicts him with claims of piety and propriety. Minutes later, a proud-looking, auburn-haired woman seated by a dark highboy starts to sing a lament. She reminds me of my Aunt Eileen, who had the same pure tone and a like touch of gray at her temples. When Sean and I were small and afraid of the dark, she would sing us to sleep with lullabies; at funerals, she sang laments that made us sad and also gave vent to our feelings.

I realize with a pang that the woman is singing my aunt's favorite, the *Caoineadh* of Dark Eileen. It opens a deep well of sorrow in my heart. I would not have it otherwise. Those who left the wild heart of Ireland carried this music in their blood as they migrated to the farthest reaches of the globe. Here, as at the source, the lament opens the door into eternity, and reveals the roots of the wild and the tame in the globe's great embrace, where we attempt to divide life into the holy and the unholy.

When the singer pauses, I take up the verses of Art's sister. I feel like a selkie who has come to this far shore to sing a soul to her long sleep. When my voice dies away, a stooped, white-haired relic of a man leans on his cane and speaks the bitter verses of Art's father. Burnt to burgundy by the harsh sun, he too—by virtue of age alone—is moving slowly into the other world.

As Reggie and I near Mr. Wheeler, we meet his vague gaze and beer-sour breath. His great bulk and bluster are useless now. He is hiding the fear of death behind drink as a toddler might cover his eyes with his hands. Reggie hugs Marilyn and expresses her condolences and then introduces me. When I express sorrow, Marilyn opens her arms.

"Nobody told me you were Irish!" she says when she embraces me. I feel at home. She releases me, and asks, "Would you sing some more? Mum's favorite was *The Shearer's Lament*."

"I'm sorry, I don't know that one."

"She liked a drinking song better, didn't she?" booms the fat, beer-swilling mourner, who has entered from the other room. In the bright light of the front room, we see that he has the leathery jowls of a rhino and a bottle of Guinness in each hand. "She'd have wanted to have a bit of the amber fluid without you lot crying in it!" He begins an angry verse of *Whiskey in the Jar* that metamorphoses into a loud rendition of *Jug of Punch*.

I feel an odd sense of comfort that he seems angry with the dead woman for escaping his control. A wake is no place for a stiff upper lip.

Marilyn ignores him and squeezes my hand. "Sing anything you like, dear."

I promise to sing another song soon, and then we follow the line and fill our plates at the table. As Reggie ladles Irish stew into a bowl, she asks, "What were you singing?"

I take a slice of firm soda bread. "That was the lament for Art O'Leary."

"It's not Danny Boy, is it?"

"It's grim. Back home, we never sang it in English because it upset my mother, especially the part about Eileen drinking her husband's blood."

"I reckon I'd rather not hear that either."

"You can't sing death a lullaby."

Reggie and I take our dinner and a pint outside to the front steps, where we sit and eat in the cool night air and peer into the dark. A breeze raises traces of soil that taste of copper and zinc from rock, and of lemon and mint from trees and shrubs. At first, my senses could only make out the boldest notes of Australia, like the cough drop smell of gum trees, the broad-brush flavors of a big Aussie red, the clamor of lorikeets, and the stony hardness of fallen gum nuts.

"Hoy, Collie! We're going to help with picking!"

Liz is running up the yard with Ronnie, who is already complaining, "I hope we don't have to see that bloody corpse!"

"How's it going?" I ask.

"Great!" Liz says, imitating my accent. "How do you like being a nun?"

"You mean a celibate? I give it four stars. I'm the calmest I've been since puberty. "

Ronnie interjects as she stomps past me, "I'm starving! Let's eat."

Liz waves, giggles, and follows Ronnie inside. I follow and continue on to the room of the departed, where several of us sing in Irish until we run out of lyrics, and then sing tunes without words. When Reggie is ready to leave, we retrace our path across the sparse grass, shuffling through the paperbark to the car. We speed in silence to the winery, holding the heavy weight of this strenuous day on sore shoulders. Reggie stops in front of the white brick house and tells me that she is going back to the de-stemmer.

I lean over to give Reggie an impulsive hug and air kiss, and then jump out, close the car door, and run lightly around the back of the car, up the sloping lawn to the veranda, and around to the rose garden, where I sit on the central bench facing the northern hills. I come here every free evening at dusk to gaze at the horizon and wonder what lies beyond. I feel permanent and yet rootless, like a nomad continuing the journeys begun by my French and Irish ancestors.

I put my arms around my shoulders for comfort, look up at the stars that spread across the heavens like fairy dust, and invite them to show me the way ahead. Thoughts arise as if in reply. *This isn't my final resting place. This much I know: I will be moving on.*

3

Randall

I stand inside the corner entrance to Flinders Station holding a sign that reads, "Randall Noll." Abruptly, the skull-pummeling sounds of trains arriving on the level below shake and invigorate the ears and bones of idle flower sellers and bored ticket takers. A surge of several hundred commuters flows up the stairs, divides into streams, and exits to tram stops in Swanston Street and to the busy streets of the Central Business District beyond.

Echoing voices beckon me to follow the joyriders mixed in with the crowd, like the tall, wide woman who is carrying a big beach bag and towing both a boy who is stamping on invisible ants and a girl in pink sandals who is trying to catch a sunbeam. I daydream that I follow and hop the tram to St. Kilda to toss up beach sand with my toes and tickle my soles on the foaming waters. If the air from Antarctica blew too fresh across the bay, I'd skip up to a sidewalk café on Acland Street to watch passersby and sip bitter black tea.

I have been feeling this holiday itch since the last grapes came in. We pressed the white varietals and drained their juice into oaken barrels, and then crushed the last of the red grapes and set them to ferment in open troughs. We celebrated the end of the harvest then and for many nights after, but our dinners felt too prim and ordered. We kept to the clock and the calendar. We passed over our need to experience the unplanned and the unpredictable. I would do that now by going to the water's edge, but Melissa's old boyfriend, who was the first to break her heart, is coming for a visit that I mean to use to create a paying holiday package and a job by which to nurture my nascent community.

A small surge of travelers ascends the shiny steps of an escalator and breaks in all directions. A man at the far edge of the white tiled floor, who has been trailing the pack, changes course and heads in my direction. As he looks up through the window over Swanston street, he smiles sweetly into the sun's rays and lowers his lids as if exalting in sensuality. He strides gracefully, like an actor on whom raggedy jeans and a bomber jacket appear to be fine men's furnishings. His forehead is high, his nose is straight, his cheekbones are brushed with bronze, and the ridge and tip of his nose are finely sculpted. As he nears, his eyes glint pure gray and his hair forms a wavy mahogany thicket that I feel an urge to stroke. A lens would love his curving lips, dimpled chin, and smoothly shaven skin, but his allure predates the camera. He could have inspired the ancients, or Michelangelo.

This time it is not only my physical loneliness that is endowing him with such allure. Other women turn to stare; one twists her heel and nearly falls. Their interest and his cat-like confidence combine to bring out the teenager in me, who still feels like a cornered mouse. He is every boy who ever dashed my girlish hopes, every man who looked right through me.

I am back at my first ballet recital. As the curtain rises, I feel the panic of exposure, and want to run away. I am in junior high school, a pimply, gangly outcast who pulls on a recital tutu and turns into a pink-fringed hot dog with no breasts and no waist. I am in high school and am, like Melissa, as sexy as silly putty. Now, she has had children with a laconic misanthrope who is at home only in the wilderness. The man walking toward me now, whose face proves the hidden harmony of the universe, whose body is the union of perfection and attraction, is a delight of creation who invites all to follow him. For all that I heard of him years ago, I cannot believe that he belonged to my old friend. Not ever. Not even for a day.

He comes nearly nose-to-nose with me before halting, flashing a blinding smile and shaking my hand. He says charmingly, "I'm Randall. Good to meet you."

His disarming smile dispels my old anxieties. Though I feel outclassed in looks and in every other aspect of worldly life, I take his hand and reply easily, "Hi, and welcome to Melbourne." As I breathe in to tell him of the itinerary I've planned, he moves on.

"I'll tell Melissa you look fine," he says over his shoulder. Words trail behind him like bubbles in a breeze as he heads for the exit to Swanston Street. He is living in a different time zone, a faster one. I rush to follow, tossing my sign in the bin as I pass, and trail him down the outside stairs and then diagonally across the busy intersection of Swanston and Elizabeth streets.

I catch up with him in front of the beautiful façade of Saint Paul's Cathedral, which stands in the iconic heart of Melbourne. Behind me is the domed yellow and brick façade of Flinders Street Station, which basks in the southern sun like a crystal palace on holiday at the beach. On the other corner across Swanston Street rises the longest-running pub in the city, where convicts, jackaroos, miners, bushrangers, police, royalists, and crooked kingmakers struck the flints that ignited the dark passions of the Australian psyche. Behind me on the right is the tram station. Beyond it, to the south, the tram tracks turn west.

"This edition of the guidebook says the Cathedral has a great view of the station and a sight line to the Shrine of Remembrance," Randall says.

As the morning crowds flow around us, Randall glances at the Shrine which rises in the distance above the westward turn of the tracks. Before he has taken time to study its gold stone prism, or the spire that points upward like the scolding finger of a forgotten man, he ticks the sight off his list. He does not pause to read that the monument's careful design admits light into the recesses of its innermost crypt only on the eleventh day of the eleventh month of the year. Armistice Day. He has not noticed that the Shrine is connected to the spiritual center of the city or to the history of Australia. Here, the First World War cut out the heart of every town, and the survivors commemorated that irreparable loss with a stone or metal monument to the dead in each town center.

Randall opens his guidebook, which is fringed with a hundred yellow sticky notes. "Let's go to the top of Rialto Towers. It has a view of the entire city."

"If I may," I say firmly, in a way that precludes further ifs, "It's still quite early and nothing's open. But I can take you on a lovely walk past several key sights."

"What walk?"

"Let me show you."

I could gesture south across the bridge over the Yarra River to the wide lawns and well-tended woods of the King's Domain, and then upward to the crenellations of the Governor General's residence and the canopy of trees that conceals a wandering chain of streams and ponds. I could mention the shy and diverse wildlife, the botanical gardens that shelter species gathered from vanishing habitats around the globe, and the formal gardens that reflect Victorian and Edwardian tastes. But first I gently pry the book from his grasp, locate a map in its back pages, and trace out the corresponding loop. "We can walk up through the King's Domain and the Royal Botanical Gardens, stop for Devonshire tea at the new teahouse, if you like, and then loop back to the National Gallery of Victoria. The Gallery should be open by then. Afterwards we could have lunch at the Southgate complex, on the Yarra River."

Randall looks at his watch and studies the book. He brightens. "Very time efficient! I have to be at Royal Women's Hospital by two."

"Ah. Well." He has made plans of his own. I make a mental note to design future tours to accommodate this possibility. "We can take the tram up that way after lunch."

"Perfect!" He gives my shoulder a pat and darts south across the street to the bridge, where he pauses to glance up the Yarra River. "Lovely."

He dashes south toward the King's Domain. I get stuck at the traffic light beyond the bridge and catch up as he plunges between the towering trees of the Domain's perimeter. I wonder if he is noticing that the trees muffle the traffic sounds and freshen and cool the air, which tastes of gum trees and grass. Before I can ask, he has rocketed up the incline toward the Meyer Music Bowl. There, he pauses on its grassy surround to view the city skyline. He puts a tick plus in the Bowl section of his book. We continue at a fast pace past a gazebo with a lovely view, lush water features, and a Japanese garden. He rushes past benches and lawns where, later in the day, lone walkers, couples, and families will rest and play.

Finally, when we reach the heart of the botany collection, he slows to evaluate hectares of specimens. In a little less than two hours, he rates a stand of old oak trees, which are too out of place for his taste and merit only a tick minus; admires the tree ferns and marks them with a tick double plus; and makes a frantic note about the damage done by the flying fox colony. Finally he gives the Australasian collection two stars.

When we have reached the southern boundary of the gardens, I say, "Let's have tea now."

"Sure thing."

When we arrive at the door of the new, glass-walled teahouse, though, we find that it is still closed. Randall folds his arms and turns impatiently away. Abruptly, he brightens and points across the placid surface of the adjacent pond. "What on earth is that?"

"That's one of the local swans. They're black."

Randall traverses a flagstone walk to stand at the edge of the water. To my surprise, he sighs deeply, drops onto a bench, spreads his arms, and commits as fully to relaxation as he did to evaluation. He knows the magic trick of controlling his state of being. In that moment, he reminds me of Reggie.

I walk to the bench and say, "I didn't think you could relax like that."

"What do you mean?" he asks without looking at me.

"You can change your state of being at will, and very quickly."

"Part of the job." He looks at me intently. I look away. He says, "No one's ever noticed. Why did you?"

I would bring up the topic of spiritual practice, but he is a friend of Melissa and a guest of the winery, so I decide to wait and take my cue from him. I drop down beside him on the uneven slats of the bench, lean back, and say, "I try to stay in the same state all the time."

I glance at him to gauge his response. He doesn't seem to notice. His gaze circles the sinuous shore, lingers on palms, plantings, and flagstones, and moves across the surface of the water, over the polo-sized lawn beyond, and up the ring of trees and urban skyline that frame the park. "Do you come here often?"

he inquires evenly.

"I've been here a few times, but I've spent more of my city time in St. Kilda."

"What's St. Kilda?"

"A neighborhood south of here. A hundred years ago it was a seaside resort, and then it declined and bottomed out in the sixties. It came back when artists moved in and revitalized it. Now it has restaurants and shops and parks. And a nice beach and a botanic garden with roses."

Randall is absorbed in the pond. I take the opportunity to study him. He is more charming than Melissa's other friends, but like them he seems a creature of hierarchy more comfortable with domination and submission than with equal exchange. It brings out my Catholic obedience. I, too, am a creature of authority and compliance—but try to make a point of moving beyond it. I put a tick minus in my mental guidebook of Randall and then remind myself that he has undertaken heavy responsibilities in his work, and resolve to make allowances for any imperiousness.

"You have gray irises," I remark casually.

"What?" he asks sharply.

"Sorry, didn't mean to disturb. I'm new to the role of tour guide." I look away in confusion. Perhaps because he is a friend of Melissa's, he is awakening my yearning for social intimacy. I feel an urge to be overly familiar, to flirt, to tease.

Randall says, "What's so amusing?"

"I was just realizing that I don't know how to be a tour guide, especially for the friend of a friend."

He gives me his full attention. "Meaning what, exactly?"

"Just now I was interfering while you were relaxing. A good tour guide wouldn't do that."

"Hmph," he says neutrally. "Melissa was wrong about you."

"What do you mean?"

"She said you'd lost your way. She sent me to check up on you. So the truth is that I'm the one who's been interfering."

We both smile. I say, "She's always been a worrier. It can be wearing, but she's the only one who cared enough about me to try and make sure I was okay. I'm lucky to have a friend like that."

For a moment, Randall envelops me in velvety attention that has the quality of a gentle embrace. His sweetly smiling eyes hold me in tender regard. I feel as if I am being seen for the very first time. When a cool breeze joins our bodies with the rustling shrubs around us, it caresses my arms. I forget about being a tour guide and savor this unexpected connection.

"Waaaaaaaah!"

A scream rises from beyond the dark green bush to our left. It has come from a tiny toddler boy who is standing alone on a gray flagstone. At his feet, a paper sack lies beside a small pile of spilt bread crusts. A black swan is swimming away from him toward an older girl. She is standing on the other side of the pond throwing fistfuls of bread pieces onto the water's smooth, black surface. Other swans and ducks turn toward her from all points, wakes converging as they dart her way.

Randall moves toward the toddler, sidles up to him and asks in mock perplexity, "Where did it go?" The boy points a tight fist at the swan.

Randall eases himself onto his haunches and teaches the tot the art of swan seduction. He takes a crust of bread and tosses it into the path of a retreating swan. A more aggressive bird spots it and swerves our way. The boy stops crying. He pumps his fist excitedly. Randall holds out a chunk of crust for the tot to take. He grips it and tosses it with all his might, sending it straight up into the air. Randall catches it and tosses it to the swan, which greedily gobbles it. Randall and the boy continue until a clot of swans converges on the tot, who is now able to offer the bread that the birds desire.

"Whoa! You're like Sandy Koufax hitting the strike zone!" Randall says

A harassed young woman appears holding a squirming baby on her hip. The baby is winding up for a big cry. "Is he behaving?"

"He's got a good arm. A born footy player."

"He's a larrikin is what he is."

"Is he a good sleeper?"

"Better than this one." She jiggles the babe while regarding Randall with suspicion. "You're a Brit, then, are you?"

"Yank. Never been to England."

Her face relaxes into a smile that's missing a canine tooth. "That's all right then. Neither have I." She takes the tot's hand and pulls him up the path. The conversation wasn't much, but it eased the woman's cares.

Randall spots the open door of the teahouse and shifts into high gear. I follow him inside and through the cafeteria line to the place where we fill our trays with the makings of a Devonshire tea, including extra pots of hot water, scones, tiny jars of jam, and petite pots of clotted cream. Randall scans the fern-filled dining area and makes for a table by a wall of windows overlooking a patio, tropical garden, and pond. He puts down his tray, takes a seat, downs a cup of black tea, opens his book, and begins to read. As I bite into a scone, I wonder if I should let him follow his book while I visit St. Kilda.

When I have watched him read for a few minutes, I say, "Perhaps you'd like to go on alone? I can give you directions and meet you at the winery."

He looks up in shock. "Why do you ask? I'm enjoying the

visit."

"You hide it well," I smile wryly.

"Just checking some facts. Don't want to miss anything."

"You're missing everything," I laugh. "We're having tea now, which means tasting it and taking pleasure in it."

"I'm that amusing?"

"I don't mean to offend. It's just that I enjoy tea and conversation. Most of my interactions are limited to sales, and I rarely get the chance to talk to Americans. I'd love to hear about your time in Sydney, what you did and how you enjoyed it."

"The research here in Australia is interesting, less regulated and more open, but with less support and fewer opportunities. They're further behind overall."

"Did you meet many Australians?"

He leans back, stretches out his legs, and puts his hands into his jeans pockets. "To tell the truth, I spent most of my time alone. I didn't feel like partying, and didn't want to spend time with expats, so I kept to myself. I intended to relax and explore, but didn't. I worked."

"Do you have work beyond today?"

"No."

I smile warmly and say, "Then let this be your time to relax."

"My turn to be frank. Why do you avoid my eyes?"

"Do I?" I am staring through the window at the lush leaves beyond. I laugh. "I guess I do. Since we're being frank, I'll confess that I can't see you when I look at you."

"Do you have macular degeneration?" he asks. He has taken me literally.

"What I mean is that I get lost in your good looks. You dazzle me. I can't see what's inside you, which means that you could be anyone. When I listen to your voice I hear the real you. I begin to know you."

"That's perceptive. I do use my appearance as a mask, for the sake of privacy. I try to do the same with my voice. I thought I had better control of it."

Our conversation is closing in on the liminal boundary between understanding and perception. I can't tell if this quick closeness reflects sympatico or carelessness. I change the subject.

"I've been tuning into voices here, noticing the way people talk of themselves. Have you noticed how many Australians in the generation ahead of us like to talk about England and Englishness? They go inside to eat hot plum pudding on one-hundred-degree Christmas Eves, and tell horror stories about the outback. They seem surprised to wake up every morning so far from home. And while they may talk about convict ancestors, they say little about colonialism per se, and it's their strongest influence."

"Like Boston."

I glance at his charming eyes, which are laughing kindly. "How so?"

"According to the book, the museum we're going to is a bluestone bunker with a waterfall, which means that it was designed to exclude the realities of geography, explicitly so when it comes to protecting paintings from the sun. Our museums are the same, and our medicine is British in its traditions, which means there's almost no difference between them and us in not knowing who, what, or where we are."

I make an uh-uh-uh sound like Grandma laughing. *Perhaps it is sympatico. He has taken me right back to the liminal boundary.* "You're right. I've been looking at it too narrowly. We're similar, especially in the European lineage, and the urban–rural divide."

"And yet different enough to gain a new perspective on

the planet."

"Yes, while we're here we see things that are new and unique, that are rooted in the land, or in Aboriginal culture. They create contrast, invite comparison."

"The Aussie psyche is intriguing."

"Especially in the way the individual psyche relates to the group-mind."

"The what?"

"The collective consciousness."

"Humph."

Now he is pulling back while I want to press on. "What do you think?"

He says reluctantly, "Shared history shapes the way people communicate."

He wants me to hold back. I take time to pour the last of my hot water on the tea leaves and to dab clotted cream on a last bite of scone. He follows suit. I leave it to him to begin again. When he does, I expect him to comment on his tea, or the weather, but he goes forward.

"If I stayed here a year, I could learn to read and imitate their signals. It would become automatic, and then I'd forget it, and come to rely on it."

He's setting a boundary. He likes the language of science. "I don't want to take any of it for granted. It can be exhausting to stay aware, but it makes experiences richer and presence deeper."

Randall grunts a reluctant assent. "So you're a mid-Pacific woman?"

"For now. I don't know how long I'll stay, but I'm enjoying it, and learning a lot about things I never noticed, or knew about."

"Like?"

"Wine's the obvious example." I frown and pause. Wine is a

world that I cannot encapsulate in words. It is held by the fields of immigrant vines, which are in viticulture around the globe; and by the crate-like cave of the tasting room, where I feel at home in the aroma of fermenting fruit; and by the winery buildings where Reggie and the others turn grapes into wine for tables near and far. In turn, these creations hold a hidden world that educates palates to savor artistry, dissolves social boundaries, and reveals the interiority of others. Rituals link these tangible and intangible elements, in ways that I am absorbing but haven't put into words. Finally, I say, "It's a way of living in harmony with nature *and* culture."

"Didn't you live on a farm before you came here?"

"A chicken farm. It was entirely different. Living there was to living at the winery like Melbourne nights are to Maine ones."

"I don't follow."

"Maine is wild in many places, a fertile interface with raw nature, a boundary land leading to infinite possibility. I didn't live in that part of it, but I was close to it and used it to create my own quiet culture at night. The winery does that for me. Melbourne at night is neon lights and raucous laughter and a clap on the back. It's rough at play, stark and dynamic at work, and it strips your psyche of protections. In that way it's like a prison."

Randall raises an eyebrow. "Sounds like they're both wild?"

I laugh. "Let me try again. On the farm, we lived at the edge of recovering wilderness, and thought of our lives there in the old-fashioned way of pioneers, as a place to scratch out a living by running a broken-down animal prison and abattoir. We feared the wild. Our lives were coarse and devoid of nuance or optimism, shepherded by the uplifting love of an exacting God whom we were brought up to fear even more than the wild. The winery is a sanctuary of cultivation and culture embraced and fed by the beloved wild. There, no one needs to go solo or hide anything."

"That's unlikely. The question is, what do they hide?"

I ponder that as I finish my tea. I don't want to bring up the fiasco at Denton, so I try to think of something more abstract and safer for both of us. After touching the napkin to my mouth and spinning my spoon in the cup, I say, "In a group, Aussies dive in without getting wet. They're open and brassy on the outside and yet guarded and secretive on the inside, as if their interconnections are so pervasive and intense that they have to conceal their innermost thoughts. So they do keep their privacy and yet they're so passionate about mateship that they'll attack anyone who threatens its egalitarian and invasive ethos." We talk about mateship and the political use of the term.

Suddenly Randall says, "What tastes are you aware of?"

"Beg your pardon?"

"You said earlier that you're always aware of the tastes, and smells."

"Ah... well, the taste of a stand of gums by a stream, or of soil minerals suspended in dry air. And the smell of herbs like lemon thyme."

"I rarely notice."

"I can take you on some bush walks near the winery, if you like."

"Yes, please. I've missed more than I realized." Randall stands. I see at the edge of my vision that he is looking at his watch.

I say playfully, "And now, we resume the speed tour?"

"You nailed it. I find it easy to turn pleasure into work."

Randall snaps his guidebook shut and clasps it in one hand as we bus our dishes. He makes an effort to move at a leisurely pace as we exit into the warming air. We cut across the park, walking side by side, talking of the change of seasons and the rhythms of the day. He points out the brown leaves that rest below the sycamore trees that line the park road, basks in the golden glow of the soaring sun, and enjoys the lull of traffic on St. Kilda Road, where we and a few idlers cross the lanes and tram tracks at our ease.

By the time we double back toward the National Gallery, which protects, or imprisons, the national art of the past, Randall's steps have become light and easy and I have relinquished the role of detached tour guide. We are making friends. At the monumental façade of the Gallery, we run playfully side-by-side along the bluestone wall, and pause to watch a wall of water run down beside the metal-wrapped glass doors. Moving as one, we enter the cool vestibule, penetrate a knot of art lovers hovering indecisively at a multistory escalator, and emerge into a lofty, brightly lit lobby. At the reception desk, a young, purple-haired girl is adjusting her fuchsia bra straps.

"We'd like to go on a tour with a docent, if one's available."

The girl stares at the place where Randall's chest hairs peek over the top button of his polo shirt. She adjusts her bra cups and then calls out, "Gracie? Can you give our international visitors a tour?"

An older woman materializes wearing a bouffant hairstyle, conservative suit, and archaic smile. She says to us graciously. "I'm Mrs. Cavendish. No one came for the early tour, so I'm available to give you a private tour of the highlights of our collection."

"No one came? So few people appreciate the importance of the fine arts!" Randall exclaims. "We're fortunate that people like you take the time to share your knowledge. Could you show us the most important international pieces? My guidebook highlights the European collection, and I don't expect to be able to visit Melbourne again."

Mrs. Cavendish smiles polite assent.

Randall adds hastily, as if remembering his manners, "And I'd like to see the Heidelberg impressionists, and Australian modernists."

Gracie gives a Queen Elizabeth nod. "The Europeans and Australians it is, and I'll also show you our special collection of Aboriginal Australian art."

We follow her into a grand old high-ceilinged room outlined in carved wood. Its walls display an Impressionist collection purchased with funds from the Felton bequest. Gracie is telling us of the time period and the painters, and also allowing us to linger at paintings we like. I am drawn toward Frederick McCubbin's "Lost," a narrow oil painting of a fragile-looking child who is wandering in a tangle of gray-green gums and tall brown grass. The child's future is tenuous. I become the child, and also the caretaker who is keen to call the Aboriginal tracker, who is the only one who can save the child.

"I've felt like that so many times! What a lovely painting!"

Randall radiates disapproval. "Rather conventional, don't you think?"

"Not in 1886! Besides, beauty is eternal."

"And in the eye of the beholder," Mrs. Cavendish adds diplomatically. "Are you two … ?"

"Dr. Noll is visiting Yarra Spur winery, and giving us the chance to try out our new weekend getaway package."

"Oh! I hadn't heard that you had accommodations."

"We're redoing the cottages and will be opening them to the public soon."

Mrs. Cavendish excuses herself to retrieve maps of the galleries for us. Randall crosses his arms and observes wryly, "I'm on the Wednesday weekend getaway tour?"

"With seder," I laugh. "I was saving a few things to tell you on the train, one of which is that my boss arranged a Passover dinner for us."

"I didn't mean to put you out."

"No, no. I'm the one who complicated your visit with a tour package, which is my way of trying to create a job here. I hope you don't mind!"

Randall smiles. "I like beta testing."

When she returns with maps and brochures, Mrs. Cavendish guides us through the European collection, which is hung in both large rooms like the galleries of a great house and intimate ones like private chambers. It mainly comprises dark oils in bright frames that I like to see as windows on the past. We look into the Renaissance though creations that reveal the beauty of humanity; and then into the Age of Exploration through visual records of the glories of nature; and then into colonial times that envisioned tame nature and high culture; and finally into wistful re-creations of ancient times. When we come to more recent works, we look into the darkness of the annihilation of nature and culture in the West, when beauty and meaning disappear, and artists see stains, hollow forms, and bitterness.

"Look at these windows into history. The collective soul has become hideous," I declare.

"They're depicting horrors that art patrons used to deny, or conceal."

"Is this what you see in the world?"

"Think of the history of the last century."

"Think of the beauties of the botanical garden, and the works of art we just viewed. If artists aid in the erasure of nature and culture, who will show what's worth restoring and enhancing?"

"It isn't always easy to see beauty, or to find meaning."

"And it's painful to abide in horror, and it's a choice."

"It's a choice to turn away from hard truths."

"And it's a choice when artists blame the world for their lack of vision." I brave Randall's gaze. "Think of Hindu religious art. It encompasses creation and destruction. These paintings are like hate speech. They're volitional, and they're destructive. They are what they purport to criticize."

Randall intensifies his gaze and smiles slyly, "In a creative kind of way."

I look away. I'd like to smile, but I have strong views on art, and find his all too common. I remind myself that his vocation forces him to face the worst and give the best, and that he has to face many horrors and to do what he can to mitigate them. Seeking concord, I say, "Nihilism can be creative if it's like the harrowing of hell, and ends in redemption and rebirth."

"You're Catholic? Melissa said something to that effect."

"I'm a former Catholic. I'm trying to come to terms with the Church, but I have a lot of forgiveness work to do. As you say, it isn't always easy to see beauty."

Randall lets his argument rest, and Mrs. Cavendish guides us back to the bright and airy lobby, which is more spacious and uplifting than many of the paintings, and inspires me to recall that we are all caught between the delight of life and the fear of death that is an eternal, insidious font of bitter horror. I try to follow my own advice of holding creation and destruction in view when Mrs. Cavendish takes us into the gallery of modern Aussie paintings and shows us Fred Williams' "Upwey Landscape."

"Brilliant! Harrowing and affecting. Very expressive!" exclaims Randall.

"Indeed," replies Mrs. Cavendish. "He painted his beloved

Dandenong Hills right after they had been devastated by a great bush fire."

"I can't like it," I add. "It's very bleak, all gray streaks and black swirls. All I know is that he was upset. I can't imagine what he lost or how he will respond to the loss."

Mrs. Cavendish exchanges a knowing smile with Randall.

"I have an art history degree," I tell him, "and I've thought a lot about the purpose of art, and chosen to make art that's useful. The art world, like literature and media, embraces problems and eschews solutions."

"You're an artist? Melissa didn't say."

"She and I don't talk about it much. I suppose she sees it as a hobby because I don't often do it for money."

"What do you do for money?"

"I'm training as a chef, but right now I'm doing whatever work I can to support my community."

"Community?"

I say evenly, "The history of the world is unfolding in each of us. We are all finding our way forward together. None of us can move ahead alone."

Randall looks at me quizzically. I am a question he cannot answer, as he is to me. Before he speaks, Gracie cuts off our exchange. She is modeling the perfect tour guide now, setting a tempo that is slow enough to engage us with each piece, and quick enough to sustain interest. She is also delighting us with variety as she opens the Great Hall to show us the stained glass windows of Leonard French, then leads us across the back lawn to see a sculpture by Henry Moore. Finally, she educates us. She takes us up the escalator past earth-toned Aboriginal bark paintings whose inscrutable dot patterns inspired the creators of decorative tourist art. We stop before an oil painting by Lin Onus, which

Gracie identifies as a piece that the museum has borrowed in the course of its preparations for a separate museum dedicated to Aboriginal art. This particular work of art is green and orange, and shows fish, a forest, and a transparent interface suggested by sinuous accents in white.

"It's like a school of spirit fish swimming in the trees!"

Randall says, "No, no. The fish are swimming under the surface of the water, and the water is reflecting the surrounding trees."

We look at Mrs. Cavendish. It is her turn to smile knowingly at both of us.

I look at the painting again. Several semi-transparent orange fish resemble swimming koi, but they are crosshatched with white patterns that are like those on the bark paintings. Lines like white ripples suggest a translucent layer at another level. In the background, lush leafy branches in strong greens suggest a forest of trees that I can't identify. The image is familiar and alien, real and imagined.

I say, "It's beautiful. And mysterious. I could stare at it for hours."

Randall's expression shifts. My body opens to his without will or understanding. We are connected in a new and deeper way to each other and to the mystery that the painter touched and revealed.

Randall remarks, "He's done it, hasn't he, pulled it all together somehow."

"What are we supposed to see?" I ask Mrs. Cavendish.

"This painting is part of a series in which the artist depicted fish in a billabong, a seasonal pond. He used white cross-hatch markings called *rak*. He was of Scottish and Aboriginal descent, you see, and he integrated his ancestry in his life and work. When he painted this canvas, however, he was not a lineage bearer entitled to use these *rak*. The elders in Arnhem Land called him to account for his actions under threat of death. People cautioned him not to go, but he went and explained his use of the sacred patterns. The elders accepted what he said and chose to initiate him into their mysteries and to give him permission to use the *rak*.

"The painting reminds me of the Celtic tradition of opening the door between worlds, but he's shown several doors of varying transparency."

Randall adds, "Or one inside the other, like *sefirot* in *sefirot*."

"Who is Sephi?"

Randall closes a mental door and erases his face. "Long story."

He reaches out to shake the hand of Mrs. Cavendish, who thanks us for our visit. We thank her in turn and descend on the escalator, exit past the waterfall window, and turn north on St. Kilda Road toward the Eiffel-Tower spire of the Victorian Arts Center. As we walk in the warm sun, my heart feels strangely heavy. I look at Randall and see from his wrinkled brow that he is troubled. I wait for him to speak. He chooses to withhold.

Randall stops at the curved entry of the Arts Centre to read a series of posters announcing the Centre's upcoming events and then bounds down the winding cement ramp leading from St. Kilda Road to the riverbank below. I take the risk of thinking aloud. "You know, meeting you is reminding me of Melissa and our old conflicts. She was willful and I was eager to please, so I let her make the choices and took the blame when things went wrong. I always expected that strategy to work and it never did. Fancy that. And now I have a tendency to see you as putting on the mantle of authority, and myself as imposed on."

"Huh." I see Randall rating me with a tick minus in his mental guidebook. "I suppose it takes a certain kind of person to take responsibility for the lives of others, even when you don't want to, and they resent it."

"You mean it's a doctor thing?"

"Yes."

"I don't know. She and I were like that as kids. But maybe that's how we came to choose our vocations."

"Or how our vocations chose us."

"Well, as you can see, I have issues that go all the way back," I say, mocking myself. "I apologize in advance for any times when I respond to my issues or to Melissa rather than to you."

"On the contrary, you're an inspiration. I've been doing inner work and I know how hard it is. When something like that comes up for me, I'm very slow to recognize it."

Randall puts his hands in his pockets. At the bottom of the winding ramp, our pace slows, and we weave through the crowds of pedestrians on the promenade. Randall scans the complex of shops and residences on our left, which rises like a temple to Mammon nestled under the spire of the Arts Centre. Randall smiles broadly when he sees the outdoor cafés at the base of the complex, where tables beckon and the gathering lunch crowd talks boisterously over clinking bottles and glasses. He inhales deeply, turns under the line of trees at the riverbank, and leans his elbows on the railing that runs along it. I join him and enjoy the view of the back of Flinders Stations and the skyline of the Central Business District beyond it.

As we watch a crowded tour boat passing under the Princes Bridge to our right, Randall says, "You know, you remind me of Melissa, too. You have that wholesome heartland look."

I laugh incredulously.

"Why is that funny?"

"Back in Maine I wore braids and overalls. When I started

working sales at Yarra Spur my boss gave me an Aussie-style makeover. I feel like a street walker!"

"Melissa always talked about you. I feel like I've known you for a long time."

"You and I have much more in common than I expected. Maybe it's through Melissa. Speaking of whom, I wonder if I could ask your advice. She and I haven't been getting along all that well lately."

"She lives in Denver and you live here. How can you not get along?" Randall jokes. He sighs and adds, "Strike that. My ex is in Houston and we don't get along."

"I didn't know you were divorced! So am I. That's what's causing my difficulties with her. She didn't want to hear about my marital problems, and can't seem to accept my divorce. I'm disappointed at her lack of faith in me, and her lack of support."

"I wouldn't say she lacks faith in you."

"What would you say?"

"Divorce upsets everyone. Especially people who are tempted by it."

"What do you mean?" It occurs to me that I may have missed the obvious. "Are you and she, um, on again?"

"Melissa has a soul mate—and it isn't me or Dan. It's John."

"John? Not the one who dumped her all those years ago?"

"He got in touch with her recently and asked her to marry him. She wanted to say yes, but she sacrificed her happiness for her family."

"I didn't pick up on it. And she didn't say," I lament.

"She didn't tell me, either. John did. He said: I used to hate you for sleeping with her, but now you're the only one who understands. He's married, too, but he and his wife live separate lives."

"How awful for all of them." A rose of shame blossoms under

my chin. "I should have sensed something was wrong. I was too caught up in my own sorry business."

"It's only natural to be preoccupied by divorce. It takes time to adjust." He adds ironically, "I'm a doctor and I'm divorced, and I haven't adjusted, so I know."

When we reach the main entrance of the shopping complex, Randall traces a curve through the crowded food court on the main level and bounds up the stairs to make a circuit of the finer restaurants. When he sees a small sushi restaurant with a minimalist black and red interior, he stops and says enthusiastically, "Let's eat here!"

"Wait!" I say, putting my hand on his arm and then pulling it hastily away. "I have to confess—I mean, I should let you know—I didn't budget for this and can't afford to pay for it out of pocket."

"My treat."

"Are you sure?"

"Absolutely. I came expecting to pay."

I catch his eye and smile slyly. "The beta test is working in my favor."

The kimono-clad hostess appears from behind a bar on our left and greets Randall with a deep bow. She leads us to a table under a circular window overlooking the Yarra River and Flinders Station. While I am still enjoying the view, she returns to take our drink orders. She promptly brings a glass of cold, plum-flavored sake and bows herself away with elaborate courtesy. Randall nods curtly. When she is gone he says, "Did you see how correctly she served the sake? Very authentic!"

"I have no idea what is correct here. I've never been to a place like this."

"Really?" he asks in astonishment, adding enthusiastically, "Perfect! I can introduce you to Japanese cuisine."

"I'd like that. Especially as I've read about the cuisine and borrowed its ideas without having tried them!"

I notice he has a *joie de vivre* that Melissa lacks, and wonder if that's the spark that drew her to him. He takes pleasure in pointing out the sushi bar and describing the training of the chefs, their knowledge of fish, and their care in its bare-handed but clean preparation. For a time we watch them dexterously filet various sorts of sea food. Randall takes me through the menu and points out his favorite raw, fried, steamed, and pickled foods. He suggests that we share plates so that I can try a variety of flavors. He is a charming host who delights in the new. I would do well to watch him closely and to emulate his manner.

After a while, when he has had his sake, and I am sipping my first-ever cup of sencha, I ask, "Do you mind if I ask you a serious personal question?"

"Ask away. I may even reply."

"It seems that you like to please people, and yet you want your own way, and expect to be waited on. Why is that?"

"No one's ever asked that!" His lips react as if he is pleased and amazed, but he does not answer my question.

"There's something else I wanted to ask."

"What's that?"

"Every now and then it sounds like you have an accent. It's subtle, but it's not Australian, or Chicagoan."

"I spent some years in India after my fellowship. It's stuck with me. Anything else?"

I smile. "Not right now."

"Just don't ask me what sex is like for gynecologists. I'm going to strangle the next person who asks!"

I laugh. "I thought you were a surgeon."

"I am. Gynecology is a surgical subspecialty. Those of us who specialize in infertility do a lot of surgery."

"You're a gynecologist who specializes in infertility?"

"That's right. I have a practice in Chicago."

I smile and look down at the surface of my tea as if sharing a joke with it.

"What is it?" Randall asks accusingly.

"It's just that I've only met two American men here, and one was a basketball player, and you're a gynecologist. I'm just wondering how many women have slept with each of you."

I glance up at Randall. He looks hurt.

"Stereotyping is such a bad habit." I say regretfully." I'm sorry I thought that, and said it."

"People don't seem to realize that gynecologists are people, too, and that our sex lives are no more, uh, interesting, than anyone else's."

I laugh. "I wouldn't expect you to know anything interesting about sex."

Randall's face turns to stone. Mine turns to ice. *Oh no, I've offended him again!*

"I've learned a few things since I knew Melissa," he says.

"Oh no, Melissa didn't say anything—" I sputter, and then I stop short when I recall her telling me that Randall was promiscuous. I gather my composure as best I can. "What I'm trying to say is that if you want to have an interesting conversation about sex, you should talk to Reggie."

"Who's he?"

"She and Andy are my community. She's my friend and boss, and the oenologist at Yarra Spur. Andy's her assistant." Seeing his cold expression, I look into his eyes and add desperately, "She's a tantrika."

His eyes transform with fascination and then fix me like a

laser. "I've heard about tantra, but never from anyone who knew what they were talking about. Is she Hindu or Buddhist?"

"Both, I'd say."

"That's impossible."

"Well, don't tell her that. She's been doing Hindu and Buddhist and Daoist practices for years."

"Does she have a consort or does she follow the left-hand path?"

Uneasiness creeps up my shoulders. I'm not sure what to reveal and, worse, my sexual centers are starting to draw energy. "You can ask her tonight. The only thing I can tell you is that she isn't a guru, and she doesn't have one."

"Do we know why she goes by Reggie?"

"Reggie is short for Victoria Regina."

"Ah. Regina Vagina. Tough nickname for a schoolgirl." Randall sips his tea thoughtfully. Gradually his face takes on a look of amazement, "That's it, then."

"What is?"

"Our commonality. Spirituality. I have a spiritual path too."

"You do? I thought you were Jewish."

"I study Kabbalah. That's mystical Judaism."

"Judaism has a spiritual path? Does Melissa know about this?"

"Yes. We've talked about it, but she hasn't studied Kabbalah. I've only just started. After the divorce I went back to Judaism, and discovered a congregation that supports esoteric practice. Do you remember the Lin Onus painting? You saw the door between worlds, and I saw sefirot in sefirot? The sefirot make up the tree of life, and each tree contains and is contained by an infinite number of other trees. Hence the sefirot in sefirot."

"That's very visual! I've heard people say a grain of sand

may contain a universe that contains other universes. But I don't recall where I heard it."

"Have you heard of fractals?"

"No."

"It's a mathematical way of expressing the idea, and it models biological systems, evolving systems, very well."

"I'd like to know more."

"What's your practice?"

"I don't really have one right now. I sit with Reggie, and read her books, but I don't have a path or a guide, so for now I'm finding my own way."

"And what are you finding?"

"It feels right to pray. I had a strong prayer practice back when I wanted to be a nun as a teen, and later as a contemplative Christian and peacemaker. But I need to pray differently now. I've been invoking Brigid, the Celtic goddess."

"Invoking?"

"Visualizing, calling on, embodying. A Jungian might say that I'm trying to understand and embody the archetype of femininity."

"Isn't Brigid the goddess of fertility?"

"I think of her as the goddess of femininity, and of cycles like the phases of the moon, and seasons, and eras and eons. And lifetimes, too; she's the goddess of maidenhood, womanhood, and elderhood."

"Are you a tantrika?"

"Only in the sense that I use the image of weaving as a model for personal transformation."

He has reopened the door between us. Our interplay is almost physical. I feel a third arising between us, and am not sure whether or how much to hold back. I look at the river and breathe into my belly to steady myself. I make sure that my sit bones are properly grounded, move my center of energy to my pelvis, and allow the infinitely complex array of set points in my body to shift. My celibacy weakens. My sexuality begins to awaken and expand; I resist, and feel the tension of resistance. I want to feel it so that I do not forget that I have a choice to make about whether to hold onto my celibacy or to let it go.

When our food has arrived, Randall introduces me to the pleasures of tempura, which he says was brought to Japan by the Portuguese, and to pickled gourd, which is sweet and earthy. I ask Randall about Sydney, and he amuses me with self-deprecating stories about his efforts to test the acoustics of the Opera House by singing during the tour, and about his bold attempt to surf Bondi Beach, which ended in a scalp laceration.

When our sashimi arrives I stare for a full minute at the glistening prisms of pink, orange, and red fish, which the chef has fringed with white threads of radish, shreds of dark green seaweed, and a perfect, bright green leaf. "What beautiful plating! But it doesn't look like food."

"Here's how." Randall takes up his chopsticks, uses them to lift a dab of bright green horseradish, and mixes it into a tiny, shallow dish of soy sauce. I notice that his hands are deft and his nail edges are perfectly groomed. "Take some wasabi. Put it in the soy, or on the fish, and then dip the filet. If you want to try the whitefish, you can add the shiso leaf for piquancy."

I follow his example and put a filet in my mouth. It is a revelation. It is submerged terroir. My tongue finds ocean and plant fire, the sea floor and the crest of a wave, purity and decay, delicacy and coarseness. I try another. "How can fish not taste fishy?"

"It's fresh. That's how you know good sushi—sashimi, in this case."

I eat slowly, delighted by each roe egg and fiber of nori. "Wasabi is better than coffee for waking up. I'm going to get some and try it on everything."

"I prefer real horseradish, with pastrami on rye. Nothing like it." Randall laughs, his lips open in delight. I try his gaze, but it dazzles and unsettles me so much that I avoid it for the rest of the meal. I talk to Randall's eyebrows, his chin, the precise corner of my shiny white plate, and the teacup marked by an imprint of the potter's hand. I begin to feel something between us that is more than casual, and wonder if it is our soul friendship blossoming, or if it is something more or different. *What pattern is this that is struggling to emerge? Do I desire him for sex or romance? Or for the kind of bond shared by Reggie and Graeme? Or for a soul friend, an anam cara?*

"Melissa said you were a farmwife, but you seem more like an intellectual."

"Now who's stereotyping? I like reading. I have an undergraduate degree in English with a second major in Art History from the University of Wisconsin, and an MFA, which means that I have a degree in passing exams, which is anti-intellectual when you think about it. Then in Maine I became a bit of an autodidact. I felt so isolated on the farm that I tried to find company by reading everything in the library except the newspapers."

"Why not those?"

"They always reflect the time-pressured state of mind of a profits-pressed editor. There's never anything new in the news."

Randall releases a soft glottal laugh and says, "I'm not averse to conventional wisdom, and I wouldn't like living away from the center of the action."

"It depends on what you think of as the center. At the winery, I live close to nature, and have soul friends, too."

"You have to make your happiness where you are."

"Which is why you're thousands of miles from Chicago?" I ask slyly.

"Good pickup. I haven't mastered it. Not yet."

An hour later, our bellies and minds in tune, we climb the ramp to cross the Princes Bridge to the tram tracks opposite Flinders Station, and there hop a tram to Melbourne University. It rolls with maddening slowness through afternoon traffic, sliding up Swanston Street like a great green and yellow eel hugging a sea floor between reefs made of buildings. Sunrays pierce the invisible roof of air, gild the gray-encrusted mass of Saint Paul's Cathedral, and highlight coral-bright shops that draw shoppers in pinstriped camouflage. At the lawn of the State Library, a thinning lunch crowd tracks the sun like a cluster of anemones. We begin to doubt that we will reach the hospital in time.

It is nearly two o'clock when we reach Grattan Street, where Randall jumps off and races ahead of me across the street and into the medical complex. I follow closely until he disappears into a maze of halls, and take a seat to wait for him in a small, quiet lobby. I close my eyes to enter the meditative state that is becoming my spiritual home.

"Colette?"

I open my eyes. Randall is looking at me intently. I say playfully, "I was just saying hi to Brigid."

Randall smiles. "My colleague was called in to surgery. We had a brief opportunity to meet face-to-face, press the flesh, make the connection. That's all I needed. We can meet again via telephone."

I arrange my clothes and purse, start down a featureless white hallway toward an exit sign, and ask idly, "Do you want to tell me about your meeting?"

"You're that interested?" he asks with a wry smile.

"I don't want to turn pleasure into work."

"I develop infertility procedures. My colleague here is trying a new method for harvesting sperm by needle biopsy."

"Oh, my."

"Madame! *Quel plaisir de vous voire encore une fois!*"

I turn to find Dr. Lee standing behind us in the hall wearing a white coat, a dangling photo id and a stethoscope. He visited the winery, and then came again several times to take me out to dinner so that he could practice his French conversation skills. He, too, is a visiting doctor—in his case from Korea.

"*Bonjour*, Lee, *ça va?*"

"Very well," he replies in French. He is wearing a wedding ring this time, and seems caught between ease and embarrassment. I am glad that we conversed—and no more. He is a reminder that the end of my marriage and the beginning of my re-acquaintance with men is a place of hazard as well as opportunity.

"Will you be in the city long?"

"No," I reply in French, with a kindly smile. "I came to meet Dr. Noll, who's visiting us from Chicago. He's trying out our new weekend getaway package." I say to Randall in English, "This is Dr. Kim Cheung Lee from Korea. He prefers to speak French."

Randall grasps Lee's broad palm and says with American pronunciation, "*Enchanté de faire votre connaissance!*"

Lee replies effusively in French. Randall's limited vocabulary runs out before he can mar any more words with swallowed a's. After we bid Lee goodbye, Randall and I continue toward the exit, where he asks excitedly, "*Tu parles français?*"

"*Oui, c'est la langue de ma mère.*"

"I'm a total Francophile. Is that how you got interested in wine?"

"Da liked whiskey, which put Maman off alcohol."

"My parents were connoisseurs of California wines."

"When we had wine, it was always French. But it was so dear that we only had it a few times a year."

"So dear? Who talks that way anymore?" He smiles.

"English majors with old parents," I laugh.

By the time we reach the tram stop, where travelers have gathered like flocking birds, Randall has extracted my family history, with particular attention to the Acadian side; obtained my opinion on the distinctions between French and Acadian culture; and debriefed me on my encounters with Lee. I wonder if he would like to ask more personal questions, but interrupt our exchange to say, "We haven't decided where we're going next!"

Randall holds his guidebook out to me in a gesture of gallant surrender. "Why don't you choose?"

I take the book. "You're a man of the book. Are sure you want to entrust it to a woman?"

His eyes crinkle. He draws closer, surrounding me in a silken cocoon of rapt attention. Time dilates. Silence gathers around. My mind loses clarity. My intentions uncoil. A packed tram rattles to a stop next to us, but I don't notice it until Randall puts his hand under my elbow and guides me gently up the sidewalk to make way for a knock-kneed young man running at the open door.

When the door whooshes shut, I open Randall's book and find a suitable map. Running my finger along a route I say, "To get to Flinders Station for the seven o'clock train to Lilydale, we can walk down Lygon Street through little Italy all the way to the Melbourne Gaol, and then take a turn to pass the Royal Melbourne Institute of Technology, which has fun architecture, and then continue through Melbourne Central to Bourke Street and the Royal and Block Arcades. If we have time left, we can stop at a tearoom there."

"What about dinner?"

"Reggie's making a Greek meal to go with her favorite big red. It should be amazing. The seven o'clock train will get us there for dinner at nine."

"Fantastic!" Randall offers me his elbow with mock chivalry.

I take his arm, and we walk side-by-side southward toward the city.

"I must confess that I had been planning to leave early and wrap up my work in Sydney, and observe Passover there, but I'd like to see more of the area. The blokes in Sydney didn't seem to think much of Melbourne, but I can see that they weren't aware of its charms."

I laugh. "There is a lot of interstate—and intercapital—rivalry. Personally, I'd like to see all of them."

"Would it still be possible to attend your friends' seder?"

"Yes, they're expecting us."

"I'd like that. I could use a real vacation before going back to the States. And I haven't seen a koala or a kangaroo."

"Can't go back without doing that! I see a visit to the Healesville Wildlife Sanctuary in your future."

4

Sparks

On the morning of the first night of Pesach, Randall and I descend from the tram to the safety zone in the median of Fitzroy Street at Catani Gardens above St. Kilda Beach. We glimpse the hues of fall that have touched Albert Park several blocks up Fitzroy, and see shoppers swarming the street's storefronts like bees in a flat, outsized apiary comprised of restaurants, fine hotels, newsagents, and fishmongers. A stiff breeze rises from the bay to tousle our hair and clothing.

In the narrow safety zone, I see a woman wearing shiny yellow Capri pants, a tight white shirt that reveals several inches of cleavage, dangly banana earrings, hot pink lipstick, and faux patent leather spike-heeled sandals. She is staring up into the tram through the door at the other end of our car, where an old lady is talking to her shopping trolley as she exits slowly. I am delighted to recognize a familiar face.

"Hi, Liz!"

Liz looks at me, and then at Randall, and chortles, "No father sky tonight!"

She winks, blows me a kiss, and disappears into the tramcar.

Randall looks at me, one eyebrow raised. "What was that about?"

"It's a long story."

"I'm all ears," he replies smartly as we dash across the street with the light.

I describe our night on the ocean beach, holding back the details. His eyes burn with curiosity. "Let's look at the high street, and then walk out on the pier and talk in private."

I point out the brick arches, cut-wood decorations, and other Edwardian details of the older buildings on Fitzroy Street, and then, as we descend to the foreshore path, I point out the green lawns and stately palms of Catani Gardens. I tell Randall about the wetlands that once flourished here, and about the development of Luna Park and the beach, and lead him through the crowds of families, couples, and teens enjoying the shore of Port Phillip Bay. We soon walk out onto the broad boards of the pier that leads a hundred yards out to a teahouse, beyond which a spit of graveled land curves to the right.

Beneath the weathered boards below our feet, white-capped waves move ceaselessly over the bottom of the bay, wearing away partly submerged boulders and sculpting the sandy bottom. To our right, fish swim in the clear waters between the shore and the spit, which embraces the Williamstown ferry tied up twenty yards ahead, and the private pleasure craft bobbing in the marina inside the spit. We have crossed the threshold into another realm. We have come to a place where it may be easier to speak of other worlds.

Seventy yards out we leave behind the ferry crew; the fishermen who have propped up their rods on the leftward rail, and who are standing sentinel over water-filled buckets; the group of elderly women in bowling club whites who amble slowly toward the shore; and the chattering group of teenaged girls in blue and white gingham school dresses and identical ponytails. When the lingering voices are lost in the sounds of the wind and waves, Randall gives me a look of intense interest peppered with impatience.

I stop and prop my elbows on the leftward rail, and look across the sparkling bay to the low granite ridges of the You Yangs. Randall props his elbows next to mine. A tunnel of attraction forms between us, carrying me back to the night on the beach. In my mind's eye, I see the four of us on the ocean beach, and then my body cocooned in the sand and sky. I recount the whole experience, including the rough times that followed, and my retreat into celibacy. When I finish, I steal a glance at Randall's face and see that it is red with cryptic emotion.

After a few minutes, he asks guardedly, "You had a religious experience through your sexual experience?"

"Does that upset you? Reggie told me not to tell anyone."

"Why would it?" Randall asks. He puts a hand around my upper arm and pivots so that we are facing each other. "Did you think it was wrong?"

"I don't know. I was taught that sex was wrong, that women were wrong."

"Look at me," he says urgently. I look into his eyes. After a pause, he asks gently, "Are you afraid of sex?"

I bow my head in confusion.

He continues, "My mother smothered me with love. My religion is sex-positive. I can't imagine how you feel." After a pause, during which I try to deepen my breathing, he asks tenderly, "Would you tell me more about the celibacy practice? If it isn't too much to ask?"

I take a deep breath and raise my eyes to his chin. "It's a Daoist practice. I breathe in and move energy within my pelvis. It's simple, and calming. It made working with Andy much easier! And now we've settled into a kind of sibling pattern."

Randall's hands slide down my arms. He takes my hands in his and waits patiently. His calm holds us. I glance up and see that his eyes are fixed on the horizon. When I feel easier he says with modulated emotion, "I felt your lack of interest in me. I had no idea that it was deliberate."

"I haven't practiced since you arrived. I feel different now," I say shyly.

I leave it unsaid that desire is awakening my sexual energy, or that my fancy is flying ahead to the formation of shared intentions and physical intimacy. I don't mention that Reggie cautioned me against this just a few hours ago, while I was telling her of the pleasure that Randall and I took in seeing the animals at Healesville Sanctuary and hiking the trails of the Cathedral Range.

"Watch yourself there, Collo," she said "He's done a bit of work on himself, but his heart's a stone, and it won't open until something breaks it open."

I was shocked by her harshness, but replied steadily. "He'd never be interested in me anyway."

"He's more than interested, and he's not as free of the past as he seems."

"Do you think it would be a problem to be with him once?"

"Sex is forever, Collie. There's no such thing as once."

"Are you saying I'll never be free of Steve?"

Reggie picks up her bag to head for the stairs and pauses; she locks my eyes with an expression of concern. "Do you think you'll forget him?"

"I think I'll become free of the emotion of the memories, with time and effort. The bond was weak, and profane."

Now, as I take Randall's arm and turn us gently back to the railing, I realize that we share a sacred bond already. We have become spirit friends through the sharing of heady ideas, and whole-body friends through physical exploration of the wonders of nature and through discussions of body and soul. We are learning to take pleasure in the delights of the day, to sense hidden troubles, and to face them together at a pace that protects our growing bond. I point out a huge white chair sculpture atop the hill at the south end of St. Kilda Beach, and then, pivoting counterclockwise, the parabolic profile of the Luna Park roller coaster; the Espy Hotel, where Reggie and I had drinks with her friends; the flat leafy suburb of Middle Park; the heavy metal rectangles that form the skyline of the Central Business District; the massive Tasmanian ferry moored at the head of the bay; the charming suburb of Williamstown; the peaks of the You Yangs Regional Park across the bay; and the place where the Bellarine Peninsula tapers off in the direction of Bell's Beach. When Randall has looked at the scene as long as he likes, we resume our course outward toward the two-story clapboard teahouse, beside which a tent-like addition is flapping noisily in the breeze.

I ask, "Is surgery like meditation?"

"It can be high adrenaline at times, but finer work, like microsurgery, takes focus, and calm."

Randall stretches his trim frame and enters into a state that is magnetic but not sexual, in which his expression is absorbed, and radiant.

"You talk easily about the body. I'm not used to that."

"You talk easily about practicing spiritual sexuality. I'm not used to that."

We walk on in silence, adjusting to a new degree of intimacy. When we reach the teahouse, we circle around to the rocky spit behind it and continue on to the cyclone fence that protects its tiny colony of fairy penguins. We grasp the wires and wait for a glimpse of the swimming birds, but see none. After a few minutes, we give up and walk back to the deck of the teahouse and look in the window. A family of five is reading the blackboard menu behind the display case. Around them, and in the tent addition on the other side, rather disheveled tea drinkers sit on rugged benches and at café tables.

As we return to the shore, the sun warms our shoulders while a bay breeze cools our legs, and our feet vibrate with the footfalls of other pleasure-seekers. When we look down, we feel as if we are sailing over the waves that run beneath the planks. When we look up, we see gulls floating on the breeze beside us as they register creaking calls and responses. The air that holds the unknown and unseen source of all embraces us, and touches our hearts with joy. Our ease increases.

I ask, "I've been wondering if Jewish sexual practices might be different than Reggie's. When she talks about sexuality she's calm and detached, whereas you seem passionate and personal. And she glows like the moon, while you shine like sunlight breaking through storm clouds."

"Storm clouds? I thought I'd been keeping my temper."

"Maybe it's just gender, but I sense tumult in you, like a struggle of dynamic opposites: light and dark, joy and anger. I think it might reflect your spiritual practice, but Reggie thinks you're still caught up in the divorce."

"She's right. You're right, too, I think. I've tried practices from the Himalayas, and they feel different. And we Jews haven't had a priestly caste since the diaspora."

Randall tenses. I feel him approach a barrier, size it up, and think about whether and how to cross it. When we have ambled another twenty yards, he takes in a breath and asks, "What did Melissa tell you about my sexuality?"

"She said that the intellectuals at your college treated you poorly because of your good looks, and that you slept with her to get access to her brilliant friends, including John."

Randall laughs. "That wasn't what I was asking but I should explain that story. I felt more for her than either of us intended. And I didn't handle it well."

"You were cruel when you dumped her. I think her feelings are still hurt."

Randall winces. "It's good we pulled a friendship out of it."

"I don't recall her mentioning anything else, except your promiscuity."

"Bingo." Randall grunts as if I hit him in the stomach and then blurts, "I always liked women, more women, new women. But I always intended to settle down and have the kind of marriage my parents did. And I did. And I worked hard at it, and managed to stay monogamous, and my wife, um, didn't."

"I'm sorry to hear it. My husband didn't, but I didn't find out until I'd left."

"She told me during a fight. Struck a square hit to the ego— on purpose, of course. We wanted to hurt each other, and got really good at it."

"I don't sense that in you."

"I'm learning to de-escalate and cooperate. She and I competed. Constantly."

"You're still in love with her?"

"I still have strong feelings about her. I'm trying for indifference. That would make this whole nightmare easier on the kids."

"You have kids?" *I walked away from my marriage. You can't do that.*

"Most people our age do."

"Most of them can't stop talking about them."

"It's a touchy subject. My ex is trying to get full custody of our two daughters. She has someone else already and wants me out of the picture."

"They'll always be yours, you know, whether she likes it or not." A hard fist of sorrow presses on the bottom of my breastbone. *You'll never be mine, not for a day, not while your heart's closed around your fear of that loss.*

When we reach the line of fishermen, Randall stops to admire a slippery, silvery fish in a white bucket, and to exchange a few words of Greek with a barrel-shaped man whose large features appear to be competing for space on his small face. Down the beach, a flotilla of women of similar age and appearance to the fishermen are undulating in the waves, watching their men. They are growing old together, and apart. That's not what I want. I want to try for a consort, or to grow old in community. Better yet, if at all possible, both.

We continue in silence to the foreshore path, where Randall stops to greet a flea-bitten shepherd dog led by an elderly woman, and a body-wagging Labrador pulling a small boy.

I ask, "Where were we?"

"We were talking about the hard stuff. Might as well finish, put our cards on the table, say what went wrong, what we regret, what we'd do differently."

"I was thinking we'd done enough for now."

Randall raises an eyebrow and looks at me skeptically. He is holding me accountable.

"All right, why don't you start? But please take it slow, give me a feel for what you have in mind."

"Ah." Randall's cheeks fill with air until he looks like the proverbial north wind. After releasing a slow breath he says, "I don't know what went wrong. Sometimes I blame our ambition, or our need to outdo each other, or the pressures of our professional lives, or the fact that each of us needed a helpmate. But I think each of us was trying to live up to impossible expectations—those of our families, and colleagues, and mentors. We took on more and more, and when it got to be too much, we couldn't admit it. We couldn't learn from experience. We thought that cutting back would mean that we had failed, and that failure was unacceptable. So we kept on going until the marriage broke. It was the weakest link, the first to fail, but if it hadn't been that, it would have been something else."

"She's a doctor, too?"

"Obstetrics. She was on call every third night."

"I think I understand. Melissa's told me about the problems of two-career families."

"Rabbi Benji helped me turn that around by meditating on the archangel of lovingkindness. Last year at Pesach, when he talked about spiritual freedom, I began to forgive. This year I'm nearly free."

"Has the custody battle gone on as long as that?"

"Yes. Lots of legal maneuvering."

"I'm trying to picture what you would have been like before. You must have changed a lot."

"Fundamentally. Instead of building a complete life that integrated my soul, I'd compartmentalized sex and love and religion and everything else. I was in pieces. It helped to open my *nefesh* to my *ruach*, and my *neshama*."

"Your what?"

"The three lower levels of the fivefold body. Flesh, feeling, and character."

"Sounds like a path to inner union."

"Yes. A difficult and slow one, but a good one."

"I'd like to know more."

As we turn onto the foreshore path, Randall says, "I'd be glad to tell you more, but now it's your turn."

"Right. I think that our deepest problem was that I never really became a woman, and he never became a man."

"Meaning?"

"We lived with his parents, and he never took charge of his life, or our lives. They suffocated him, and he crushed me. We never came of age individually or together. When we didn't have children, we became the children, and our bond was never strong, nor sacramental. We expected the marriage to happen by itself. We relied on the early romance to carry us through. We didn't face the problems or do the work."

"The good thing about divorce is recovering personal responsibility, giving up the cycle of blame." He asks carefully, "Will you ever remarry?"

"I don't know. It isn't my first priority."

"What is?"

"Giving birth to a community, and finding a consort."

"A consort?"

"Someone who wants to be the partner of my life work, to father something that will make the world a better place."

"Not a child?"

"A spirit child, or a brain child. A shared vision that leads to purposeful, meaningful action. That makes good on our past and makes the best of our skills and opportunities."

"That's beautiful, compelling. My colleagues and I ensure human fertility without thinking or talking about what it is or what it means."

When I hear our words, they penetrate the part of my mind where patterns reside. Shapes shift like shadows beneath a tree illuminated by the piercing sun. Where my mind's eye found chaos and shadows, it sees a new form emerging. I feel a third taking shape, a fresh presence with a life of its own. In my heart, a bleb of festering feelings breaks open, inviting me to cleanse its bitter juices.

I say with unexpected force, "My marriage was dead, spiritually and sexually. It was like a perpetual crucifixion without a resurrection. I want to cleanse myself of it inside and out. I want to bring my body and soul back to life, and I think the best way to do it is to practice sacred sexuality. That's why I hope to find a consort who will synergize with me instead of antagonizing me."

Randall looks shocked. I must have penetrated old pat answers, and hit him unexpectedly hard. I add with light irony, "Aren't you glad you asked?"

He stops in the middle of the path. A cyclist nearly collides with him. "I feel that way too. I can't bear to think of how it was. I want to walk through the fire. I want to burn it all away. Every expectation, every trace of thwarted rage."

When he begins walking again, I say, "When we put the past to rest, we'll be able to behave as if the best is yet to come. Okay? Enough hard stuff?"

"For now."

Strangely tired and slow after our emotional exertion, we continue our southward stroll. I point to the beach and tell Randall how it was in summer when nearly nude sunbathers covered the machine-groomed sand, and red-hatted members of the St. Kilda Life-Saving Club scanned the water for struggling swimmers. I describe the traffic on the foreshore path, which was heavy, and point out the old baths that have been closed for years; the Palace that is host to rock concerts; the palm-lined Esplanade where the arts and crafts market convenes on Sundays;

the playground that was filled with preschoolers; and the scenic railway—a roller-coaster—encircling Luna Park that sent up screams of mock terror.

Randall remains polite but preoccupied.

"So, what happens at a seder?"

Randall tenses. "That depends."

"Is it like a Mass?"

"It's a meal to commemorate the Passover."

Randall stops again and regards the golden sandy beach, which holds a smattering of sunbathers and sandcastle builders.

"Is everything all right?"

Randall sighs. "What do you know about Judaism?"

I rummage through the attic of my mind like a coin collector looking for steel and nickel pennies. I find only slugs: celebrity gossip, like Bob Dylan's conversion to Christianity; Yiddish words like yenta; and food facts, like a good bagel should be boiled before it is baked. And then I find a penny thought. "Melissa said it was hard being married to a Jewish man. Their kids didn't seem to fit in anywhere until they had their *bar mitzvahs*."

Randall objects irritably, "It doesn't have to be like that!"

"Holidays can be difficult after divorce. We don't have to go if you don't want to."

"I want to! It's a high holy day for me. But it isn't easy. It raises difficult memories. I came to Judaism through my grandparents, who fled pogroms in Eastern Europe and then lost family members in the Holocaust. They were happy to celebrate a vengeful deity that killed other people's children. I wanted to get away from all of that grief and hatred. I left the tradition for years. And then when I found my way back, my wife took the children—I have visiting rights only, and at her convenience—which means that I can't pass on the tradition as I have come to know and love it, which is what a seder is for."

"What is it that you would pass on?"

"I'd share the joy of honoring the past while creating a living tradition that evolves with human understanding. Some think of observance as obeying laws, of which there are 613 in the Torah alone. But we can understand those so-called laws as principles that take on new life and meaning every year."

"Are you saying the Old Testament is changing?" I ask incredulously, my Catholic habits awakening and obscuring my growing belief in continuing revelation.

"Life is always revealing new ways of understanding ancient texts. Think of how I've ended up here at Reggie's winery, talking with you about sacred sexuality. It's a sign. I want to read it, and understand it, and use it as a guide for continually refreshing the living covenant."

"Your arrival does seem like a harmonic convergence or something."

Randall brightens and says eagerly, "Coincidence is our recognition of possibility."

"Possibility?"

Randall's eyes search mine. I feel his breath on my upper lip. The world contracts around us until we seem to be alone far from the waters of the bay in company with a silent question of great weight. Randall says gently, "Do you see any possibilities in me?"

Sadness pushes its fist against my chest. I don't know if the sensation is his or mine, or both. "I saw more before you mentioned your children."

He smiles almost imperceptibly. "Are you sure?"

"I'm not sure of anything."

I look away, take his elbow, and guide us onward. The moment is full of silent questions that cannot be put into words, that break through old forms. I no longer know what is easy or hard, right or wrong, a sign or a coincidence. Everything seems made of quicksilver: heavy, but fluid and changeable. After a time, when we reach a restaurant that sits between Luna Park and the fore-shore path, I ask, "Shall we have lunch?"

"Sure."

We circle the gray wooden building and enter the front door. A trim hostess greets us and seats us at a table on the patio beside the beach. Our chairs touch a white chain that separates the patio from the bike path. When a bareheaded cyclist whizzes by he touches us with his airstream and sends a nearby roller-blader and baby stroller onto the cement walkway beyond. A party at the next table issues a verbal editorial on the errors of careless cyclists.

Randall leans toward me. "It's strange to celebrate Pesach in the fall, even if it is a harvest festival in Israel."

"It was wonderful leaving Maine in winter and coming into the southern summer."

"Don't you miss Maine?"

"I miss a few things, like the Acadian fêtes. Last year my brother came up from New Orleans to play his fiddle, and I sang with him, like when we were kids."

"Do you plan to return?"

"No. And yet I don't expect to stay here for the rest of my life."

"Do you want to?"

"I feel like I haven't found the right place yet, but that I'll know it when I find it."

"I thought you were going to be a tour guide," Randall says cheekily.

"It seems that I lack the requisite detachment. Maybe I've absorbed the Aussie spirit of play without learning Aussie rules."

Randall smiles crookedly. A black-eyed waiter with jutting cheekbones and a hollow chest takes our drinks orders, after which Randall and I take turns to go inside and read the fluorescent pink and green menu on the mirror above the bar. While he is gone, I scan the beach for the sculptor who built castles here in the summer, but the blank beach has now become a canvas for the long, low waves that are painting undulating lines of seaweed and shells.

When Randall returns, and the waiter has brought our drinks and taken our orders, I ask, "What about you? Are you looking forward to going home?"

"I'd like to bring some of this with me, the sun, the élan."

"You're not looking forward to going back, then."

"No, not at all. My senior partner, Stan, is like a second father, and my junior partner, David, is like a little brother. We're close, very close, but the divorce has poisoned the atmosphere. It's been rough on Stan and Ellie, and David's wife took my wife's side. I love them, but the truth is that I've been thinking of selling my part of the practice. I want to move on."

"Your situation is very complicated. I wish you all the best."

"Thanks. You've been a real inspiration. I admire your courage. I've never liked taking risks, and now that everything's so uncertain it's harder, not easier."

"It's different when you have kids. Take Abraham. He could leave everything he knew because he didn't have kids."

"Until he and his wife were old." Randall puts down his fork, looks at me intently, and asks with careful carelessness, "What made you say that?"

"Say what?"

"How did you happen to think of Abraham?"

"I don't know. I suppose it's your talk of the Torah."

"I've been thinking of Noah, and Moses, and Rabbi Akiva, but I haven't thought about Abraham for some time."

"And?" I ask in puzzlement, and then, seeing the keen expression on his face, I add, "Is it a sign?"

"Ask me next year, after *HaShem* creates the world again."

"Beg your pardon?"

"I mean when we return to the part of the Torah that tells of Abraham, which follows the story of the creation."

"I'll send you an email. If I can figure out when that is."

Randall laughs. The waiter brings our plates. I spear a sun-dried tomato and savor it. The calm of celibacy is declining, and all of my senses are opening. The taste of the tomato fills my body with deliciousness that awakens pleasure in my skin. I say, "This is so amazing! You're welcome to taste one. I'm sorry I ordered bitters, now. These tomatoes would be wonderful with a big Aussie red."

We natter about food and wine, enjoying the sun and bay breeze, and the jovial mood of the other diners. Gradually, we let weighty topics drift away, and feel free to enter into the spirit of the foreshore, which is different from that of our themed excursions in the Yarra. We have the chance to play with spontaneity, to try choices that carry little weight like ordering an unfamiliar lunch, eavesdropping on conversations that form windows into other lives with other cares and joys, and talking on tangents.

For a while, Randall speaks of his work. He loses me in a tangle of tubules, but seems to be talking something through, and so I listen and wait patiently for understanding, or for him to move on. After a while, when it becomes clear that he, too, is ensnared in his endless cycle of detail, I draw his attention to our empty plates, and we resume our walk south on the foreshore path. When we reach the marina, we turn away from the bay and walk along a residential street to a long grassy park. We are like tourists now, walking north across the park to a large oval, where a low cement clubhouse building displays a small sign indicating its affiliation with the St. Kilda Football Club. We lean on the board fence, which corralls the oval, and watch clusters of men and boys play footy inside.

A few yards in, a group of schoolboys take turns running up the back of a ruddy, thick-necked Atlas. One boy makes it to the man's shoulders, perches there, and throws the flattened ball. A man, possibly his father, dives to catch the pass. At the far end of the oval, a few trim players wearing a colorful mix of jerseys kick a ball back and forth. In the middle, a few men with thick bellies struggle to reenact youthful glories. The scene is a clan of Scotsmen, a mob of Blackfellas, or a Connolly family reunion— everyone playing at once, and each in his own way.

We walk on to Acland Street, where we stay under the awnings that shade the shop fronts and pause to admire the sculptures that rest on the roofs of the metal awnings across the street. One's a colorful rock band, and another a missile that has the tail above and the tip below. I tell Randall of a supposedly secret American base in the outback that planted an errant missile outside William Creek Pub. Passersby smile with me, but Randall is not listening.

He doesn't want to go back. He is looking for someone. This could be more than a fling. I tell myself not to get my hopes up. I remind myself that he has not said that he is looking for a consort, or a partner of any kind.

"Look!" Randall says excitedly. "A book shop."

"Yes, it's my favorite."

Randall speeds past cake, fish, and clothing shops to enter a narrow shop lined with floor-to-ceiling shelves. I follow. We stand together in the entry until our eyes adjust, and we see that the store is filled with quiet browsers. I lead Randall to a few dark and raucous novels by Aussie writers, and then to a section of children's books featuring bush animals like bilbys and quolls. When he has chosen a few, and is waiting in line to pay, I notice that sunset is approaching.

"We should catch the next tram," I say.

Randall nods. His expression is grim, and remains somber as we join the rush hour crowd that is waiting at the open-air depot across from Luna Park. The trams are frequent now, and the Friday afternoon crowd seems dominated by frazzled workers who are going home, and revelers heading to parties. We wait in silence for our ancient yellow and green car to stop and then squeeze aboard before it heads east, away from the water. We cling to its yellow metal posts until we reach St. Kilda Road, where we descend and change trams. When the next tram has screeched and clanked around the corner into Glen Huntley Road, Randall suddenly gasps and pushes his way to the door to peer out at something. The other passengers make way, wary of his distress.

"What is it?" I crane my neck and glimpse a white-lettered sign that points the way to a Holocaust Memorial.

Randall grips one post and then another to peer excitedly at the busy sidewalks, where many pedestrians are wearing black hats and ear curls. When the doors open at the next stop, Randall unexpectedly jumps off. I push through the crowded aisle of the tram and manage to clear the doors before they close. He is already a block away. I finally catch up in front of a kosher butcher shop, where he is staring at the glass above an open door.

I follow his sightline to a saucer-sized white spider that is clinging to the glass. "Don't worry, it's only a huntsman. They're not poisonous."

"It seems to be guarding the door," Randall says suspiciously. "As if it's defending itself, or as if it feels vengeful."

"Maybe it's a Rorschach spider," I tease gently. "Maybe it takes on whatever patterns and meanings you project on the world."

Randall smiles distractedly. His notice of me is dissolving, or disappearing behind a force field of feeling that he is erecting between us. He swivels and heads farther east at a brisk pace. At a bakery window, he stops abruptly, grabs my arm, and whispers urgently, "Do you see his arm?"

Inside, two men are sitting opposite each other at a table. One is short, slender, and dark-haired, and though his back is toward me, I can see his bare arms, which are forming an upside-down V around a foamy cappuccino. On one arm I can see an irregular, hand-written blue number. The man's companion is bald, and his face is strangely unmarked by age. When he lifts his arm to take a drag from a cigarette, I see a similar blue number.

"I see numbers."

Randall grabs my arm. He drags me past shops and restaurants to the nearby corner, where he stops abruptly and asks hotly, "And do you know how those numbers got there?"

"Did I do something wrong?"

Randall's tension eases slightly. "It isn't about you."

I pry his fingers away from my arm. "Steve used to blame me for things. I did it too. I want to be on your side, but you can't take things out on me."

Randall hesitates, and then plunges into a hell state. "They're concentration camp numbers. They were written by the Nazis over fifty years ago!"

He turns in the wrong direction. I reach out, hook his arm, and guide him gently across Glen Huntley Road toward Hal's home. Glancing now and then at Randall's discomposed face, I recall Reggie's warning. His heart has closed around the loss of his marriage and family and the unbearable events of history. The former I can meet with understanding and equanimity; the latter baffles me. I have no idea how to act as a consort to a man whose heart has been stamped—however indirectly—with unspeakable violence.

As we walk, the past rests on our shoulders like a pack filling with rough weights that deepen Randall's angry sorrow, and lead him to personalize and perpetuate the effects of cold, efficient genocide. I have seen him respond that way to reminders of nuclear devastation, habitat erasure, and addiction to consumptive destruction. These weigh down our species, and yet I have learned to leave those weights by the wayside as I take up that which I choose to change. Now, to support Randall, I try to do that with him, and so become his consort for the day.

I try dark humor. "Can we talk about your divorce again?"

Randall snorts. He has heard me. I am breaking through.

I take his arm and stop. "Look at me."

He bites his lip. He shakes his head. And then he looks, and does not look away. "Our marriages were hell states of cold and heat. Since divorcing, we've experienced heavenly states. We felt them today."

"And?" he replies impatiently.

"There's no virtue in residing in a hell state. Wouldn't you agree?"

"What's your point?"

"Tonight, let's be Brigid and Solomon, let's celebrate the perpetuation of life, and of love."

A trace of a sardonic smile touches his lips. I kiss them lightly.

"Solomon, eh?"

"The one with the hit song."

For a minute, he remains tense, and then he relents and sighs. "The Song of Songs. I don't have to dance?"

"The hora?"

"You do know about Jewish life!"

"I went to Melissa's wedding. And sometimes I remember bits of it."

Randall whispers, "*L'chayyim.*"

"And later, when the time is right, I'd like to hear more about the world healing you talked about yesterday. I'd like to try it, too."

"*Tikkun olam.* The practice of practices."

When we reach the residential street where Hal lives, we pass a huge kindred walking together. Most of the men are wearing ear curls, black hats, and black suits topped with tasseled shawls. When they have passed, Randall tenses and exclaims in the anguished tones of a cornered man, "I never guessed that Reggie's friend might live in a neighborhood like this! We could be in the Warsaw ghetto. It could be starting again."

I take his arm. When we reach the street corner, I stop under a fragrant gum tree and gesture toward the shady cross street, where blocky, modern homes have replaced Edwardian ones. "We're in Melbourne. It's a beautiful fall evening. We're on our way to Hal's house to share in his family's dinner. The people around us seem loving, and expectant, and joyful. We're far from Europe, and it isn't happening again. What happens next is up to us."

Randall nods and sips a raggedy sigh of menthol-flavored air. "I'm sorry. I thought I was ready for this."

"I get upset whenever I go into a cathedral, especially a beautiful one. I have a hard time remembering that I don't have to say yes to all of it, that I'm free to do what I think is right."

"It's hard to be grateful at times."

"And to let the wounds heal. We can confuse old wounds with sacred obligations."

Randall gives me a penetrating look, and then gestures for me to lead. He seems glad of my company. I begin to believe that I have what it takes to steady him, perhaps even to bring out the best in him. The knots of our hearts may have been tied by different hands and in different ways, but they are enmeshed in the same threads of time, and hold the same urge to loving union.

By the time we reach Hal's house, which is made of smooth, brown bricks, the sun has sunk behind the trees, and we are breathing easy. I stop and say, "We're here. Do you want to go in?"

Randall takes something out of his back pocket, unfolds it and pins it into his wiry hair. It is a silky white yarmulke. "Yes, thanks."

5

Improvisation

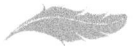

hen the door opens, family tension spills out and takes
hold of us like a mean-drunk host who whispers nasty
nothings in our ears. It is a shock to see Dutchy's petite blond
beauty marred by matted hair, angry eyes, and pressed-white
lips, and to see her feelings vented by the bald, squirmy baby
who is trying to wriggle out of her arms above the entry tiles.

"Hi, Dutchy! This is Randall, our visitor from the States.
Unfortunately, Reggie couldn't come with us. Thanks so much
for—"

"*Chag sameach.* Come in!"

Dutchy disappears. We enter the white, minimalist interior,
where we see her collapse onto a tweedy couch, pull out a vein-tat-
tooed breast, and try to soothe the baby with milk. Her accent
is unusually heavy with esses as she explains to us distractedly,
"Hal iss very upset. Hiss mother hass just now decided to have
seder with the little brother, who iss rich."

"It's always so difficult when—"

"And after sseee bullied me for yearss to be blooded!"
Dutchy adds.

"Blooded!" I exclaim in shock.

"When a woman hosts her first seder for the family, we say
that she hass been blooded," Dutchy explains. We hear a metal
pot clatter on the floor in the neighboring kitchen. The baby, who

is like a tuner broadcasting his parents' distress, emits a wobbly-lipped scream and tries again to fly over onto the hard wood floor.

Randall plops down beside Dutchy, utterly relaxed. I remember what he said about relaxing during surgery, and suspect that he is in 'doctor mode,' as Melissa calls it. "How can we help?"

Dutchy pushes a pacifier into the baby's mouth. He pops it back out.

"Do you want me to take him for a while?" I ask. "I have thirty-one cousins, and had a hand in bringing up most of them."

"I can help, too," Randall offers. "I have two daughters."

Dutchy allows me to take the baby and watches as I turn his back to my belly, where he can see her, and then move slowly back and forth, humming and jiggling. The baby quiets.

"What's his name?" Randall asks.

"Jossie," Dutchy replies warily.

The doorbell rings. Dutchy points us toward the baby's room and goes to greet her guests. Randall and I walk down a narrow back hall to the nursery, where the baby's demons engage us. We have no thought but to soothe him. We change his diaper, offer pacifiers, and try every other distraction we can devise. We take the baby in turns to circle the room, and then go up the hall past the kitchen, where Hal is still struggling at the stove. We move on through the dining room, which is already set for dinner, and then back to the nursery. We avoid the living room, which is filling with guests who are sharing the drama of distress. A long half hour later, Randall has calmed the baby by dangling a shiny pendant in front of his eyes.

One by one, our hosts and their guests come to see the baby and to share the gossip. Within an hour, they have painted a word portrait that tells as many tales as Rembrandt's Nightwatch, and we understand that the fabric of this family is torn and may never be patched. Before today, Hal had taken for granted his position in his family. He was the oldest and smartest, gained pride and security through his position as a renowned professor, and enlisted his mother's help in teaching Dutchy to be Jewish so that their baby could also be. Hal's younger brother, who was less gifted but more ambitious and canny, established a chain of mid-priced clothing stores that enabled him to buy a grand home in the posh suburb of Toorak. All went on as usual until today, when Hal's sister-in-law, her family, and their rabbi persuaded the mother that because Hal was strictly secular, Dutchy had not really converted to Judaism, and their baby would never be Jewish. The balance of power shifted, and the younger brother took the place of the elder. The mother could not bring herself to speak to Hal, so the brother called to break the news.

"Do you think the baby is Jewish?" I ask Randall.

"I think a person is Jewish when they do the work: make the choice, study the teachings, unify the body, and return to *HaShem*."

"I wish there was another word for we, one that meant all of us. Did you notice that Dutchy said we, meaning that her baby's Jewish? Her mother-in-law's going to use the same word to mean he isn't."

Randall nods, and shrugs with his eyebrows. We stand face to face, the baby and his uncertain future hovering between us. Before today, the mother shaped Dutchy and her expectations, and insisted that Dutchy undergo a gantlet of trials by which her baby would be included in the family we. Now, through his aunt's gerrymandering, the baby has been cast out of the warm love of we and into the cold suspicion of they.

When the kitchen has filled with helpers, and the doorbell has not rung for ten minutes, Dutchy calls us to bring baby Jos to the dining table. We come and put him in his high chair, and take the available seats, which are on opposite sides. Dutchy, who is seated beside Jos, is red in the face. Hal rushes in from the kitchen to take his place at the head of the table, his face purple with pent-up emotion. The baby begins to cry miserably again. The veins on his fuzzy scalp bulge blue. It seems that someone at the head of the table may explode.

Randall says charmingly, "I wonder if I might say a few words as the traveling guest?"

Hal gapes in surprise. Someone at the other end of the table begins to object. Randall raises his palms to signal silence. I look from his hands to his radiant face. On the wings of memory, I fly back to a hike that he and I took above the stringybark forest of the Cathedral Range. We are on the last arduous stretch of the Ned's Gully track to the summit of Cathedral Peak. We are hot and tired and exhausted. My hamstrings clench like fists. Each step raises dry dust and bitter thoughts. I have pushed my body too far—it is running on anger.

In the middle of the last monotonous steps up the crumbling sandstone, as I watch Randall's dusty calves pump like those of a leadout in the Tour de France, he halts abruptly. I narrowly miss bumping his sweaty backside, and have to catch my balance. When I wrestle my eyes away from the precarious footing, I see that Randall is taking in the panorama from the fecund expanse of the Acheron Valley to the crumbling crest of Mt. Sugarloaf. When he turns to extend his hand, his glowing eyes fill me with joyous kindness. The efforts of the day burn away; vitality returns. And then his soft, strong hand lifts me into a state of being that is not spiritual or sexual or any one thing. It is complete. It includes all that I could want.

Now, Randall's eyes sparkle as he says, "I want to thank you for opening your beautiful home to us on this night, which is different from all other nights, and to say that Colette and I are especially honored to be at this Pesach seder, which is different from all other seders because it is your first as a father and the first of your firstborn son in your family home."

A wave of emotion passes down the table. Randall has broken the hold of fretful unhappiness. He has brought something of heaven to earth, and let us all touch the sacred. Hal buries his face in his napkin and feigns a fit of coughing. Seeing Hal overcome by emotion, Dutchy creates a distraction by springing from her chair, extricating baby Jos from his, and asking in her thickest accent yet, "Does everyone have de wine, and de parsley and salty water? And be sure you haves some of de wasabi and arugula and dip!"

Randall asks, "Wasabi? Dip? Are these local traditions?"

"Dey are part of diss new expression of the tradition dat we made for you."

A murmur goes around the table. I wonder what the group expected, and what Dutchy has done differently. Each of us has a round plate unlike any I have ever seen. Its radial array of egg-shaped depressions each holds a different tidbit. Dutchy explains that each item represents an aspect of the Jewish experience of slavery. By the time we confirm that we have what we need, Hal is ready to preside over the dinner. He blesses the wine in Hebrew, washes his hands, and instructs us to dip our parsley in salt water. Randall is one of the few guests who has the ritual by heart, so I imitate him. When we have dipped our parsley, we wait as Hal says another blessing and then eat the parsley. Then Hal breaks a matzoh and hides part of it for the youngest to find, after which he looks at Jos as if hoping for a leap in maturity.

Dutchy hands out copies of the Haggadah, and those who are

literate in Hebrew take turns reading its passages out loud. There is an English text so that the rest of us can follow the telling of the Jewish people's exodus from Egypt. Hal calls this story the Maggid, and says that it is passed from one generation to the next through the family, and that it is designed to engage family members of all ages. At first I enjoy the story, which assumes that even the smallest child knows the Sabbath ritual, and how this one differs from it, but I notice the word "we" appear again and again like a sentinel set out by long-gone priests.

It is a magic word set like a seal in the mind, creating boundaries of identity that draw on the oldest sources of power: demonization, taboo, cursing, and scapegoating. The magic word "we" pulls me back into the promise of security that is enforced by visiting violence on seeming enemies, and by joining fear to hatred to create a force that can rise and break with the power and speed of a tsunami. This security can take forms like war and culturcide, as befell Jews like Teresa of Avila and Druids like the Irish priestess Brigid, who were coopted into sainthood.

The nuns taught us that Jesus loved his enemies as himself, but few showed us how to live that teaching. My eyes fill with tears for love of this promise and for regret at its lack of fulfillment in me. *I still have a chance. I've already changed.* I no longer feel the pull of saintly suffering spiced with the hot and sour flavor of sadomasochism. Saints made glorious by a vengeful father God no longer raise my sympathetic agony; nor do images of substitutionary sacrifice comfort me when I err. I have escaped conformity to arrive in the no-man's-land between boundaries—the same place where Dutchy is wandering, the place of the universal outsider who wishes to be enemy to none but becomes "they" to every "we." The clerics and vigilantes who patrol this zone fear us. We remind them that their boundaries are imposed, and thus subject to loss or transformation.

I look to Randall now, and dote on his glowing love for his tradition with all its human flaws. His love does not appear to exclude me, or anyone; like Reggie's, it seems to be exemplary in its inclusiveness, to be free of boundaries that pull love inward by pushing aversion outward. I knew nuns like him, whose hearts were so filled with love for all creation that it illuminated every shadow; their love forgave all wrongs, including those of their beloved church. This kind of love stays true to the unfolding search for a sacred trust that welcomes all living entities, tangible and intangible. This love is the love that I would wish for us all to feel, now and later, together and apart. If Randall, too, wants this love, I could steady him in this borderland, and he in turn could steady me.

When the Maggid is finally finished, the guests in the know go to help with the feast, or take time to introduce themselves. After that, the twenty faces around the table focus on food and family. The shy, balding man sitting beside me reminisces about the seders of his childhood, recalling with fresh glee the time that he was the one to find the hidden piece of matzoh. On learning that Randall is newly single, a stocky, dark-haired man sitting nearby criticizes Dutchy's tzimmis recipe, compliments Hal on his first attempt at gefilte fish, and says that the matzoh balls are a fine first try but cannot compare to those made by his single and available sister, a plump woman at his left. He asserts those are so light that they float above the soup.

Others, like me, who found the Maggid grim and unloving say little, and then fall silent. Among these is a cousin of Hal, Saul, whose lined face became a tragic mask during the Maggid's ponderous tale, as if its telling had enslaved his tribe all over again. Soon Saul falls back into the mood that prevailed before Randall spoke to the group, and quells the delight that had resurfaced by asking Hal to talk about his mother's choice. Hal and Dutchy slouch in discouragement. Hal shakes his head and says nothing. The baby becomes inconsolable. The group skims over the grace and the psalms and then lifts their glasses as one to say, "Next year in Jerusalem!" their voices creating an uneasy mix of fervor, sarcasm, and strained politeness.

Hal says edgily, "Well, that's it, then, unless the doctor rabbi has anything else to say."

"Actually, I do. I want to thank each of you for your part in creating this wonderful seder, which has reminded us of our shared past, and has even brought it to life again. When Colette and I arrived earlier, I was surprised to find that you, Hal and Dutchy, live in a neighborhood that includes so many Orthodox Jews. I could sense my dead father beside me, who longed to belong, and yet was so secular that he would argue with anyone who said so.

"I think of the Nederlinkatz grandparents who fled Eastern Europe and took the name Noll at Ellis Island, and were so strict that their children became leftist agitators. I think of the wealthy Stein grandparents, who did something mysterious during Prohibition. I picture the father with whom I reconciled just before his death, the aging wisp of a mother I still adore, and the brother who broke down and exiled himself to a strip of sand off the Florida coast. I try to imagine what came before, and what may follow.

"I came back to Judaism for the path of healing. I intended to heal my patients, but found that I could not heal them without also healing myself and the world. This is obviously a task for many lives and lifetimes, and for many beings, including the angels and the One with whom we wrestle. Tonight, I feel renewed in that task. Meeting people like you, who offer shelter to the stranger, and who set such a beautiful example of blessing, helps me on my way. I trust that it helps all of us on our respective ways, and I think I speak for all of us in saying to you, Hal and Dutchy, thank you for sharing your home, your blessings, and your community."

"Amein!" adds a tiny, sprightly man at the foot of the table.

"Thank you, Rambam!" says Hal cheekily, his mood lifting.

Randall's manner has been so charming and his energy so beneficent that I take in his words like an after-dinner liqueur that dulls the sharp edge of reality enough for me to once again imagine the errors of the past slipping away, and the tribe and species moving smoothly on to a better future.

The group rises. Chairs scrape against the floor as if removing the residue of a year of servitude. Half of the guests go to the living room to talk and the rest go to the kitchen to help. As Dutchy extricates the baby from his high chair, I ask, "Do you want us to take the baby again?"

"Yes, pleasse!"

Randall and I take Jos back to the nursery, where I sit in a white rocking chair. Randall rests the baby on my breastbone, and I start to sing my favorite Scottish lullaby, *Dream Angus*, in my lowest register, so that the notes resonate through my chest and into the whimpering Jos. Randall looks around the room for a place to make his own and lies down on a huge sheepskin rug. I close my eyes and feel the warm, soft weight of the baby and think of Randall. As Jos grows quiet, I drift on to snatches of love songs in Irish.

When Jos is asleep, I open my eyes to see Randall looking at us, and whisper, "I so enjoyed what you said, but I didn't like the Haggadah!"

Randall laughs. "A terrible choice for this family! I wish I'd brought mine."

"Yours is different?"

"You can look at the story of Passover in many different ways. We see Torah as the story of human consciousness. As we evolve, we find new meanings in the past, which means that our interpretation changes every year. Without that, the tradition dies."

"How does yours differ?"

"Today I would say that the Jews knew the plague was coming, and tried to warn the Egyptians, but the Egyptians didn't listen."

"What about the God who killed so many Egyptian children, the ones who weren't slaves, and weren't passed over?"

"I don't know. It could mean that God found slavery unacceptable, and had no other way to end it. Jews lacked the skills of non-violent action. We've tried it time and again, as early as two millennia ago, but non-violent social change didn't come into being until much later, through Tolstoy and King and Gandhi."

"I'm glad you said that. I don't like tyranny, theocratic or otherwise."

"My rabbi is a teacher, not a tyrant. He listens, learns, and forms opinions, but he doesn't force them on others, and doesn't pretend to speak for *HaShem*. He argues with angels and with *HaShem*, though; we all do."

"Argue with God? I'm glad the nuns can't hear you."

"We don't see human beings as passive participants in creation. We don't see ourselves as beasts of spiritual burden. Not any more. We're partners who bring everything, even God, into question. The way you might try to be like Brigid, we try to be like Jacob."

"Not Solomon?"

"That one's new to me. But I like it," he says with a mischievous smile.

"I could never convert to or follow any religion, not after how I was brought up, with tyranny and hierarchy and damning everyone else to hell."

Randall observes, "Maybe it's for the best."

"What do you mean?"

"Obstacles force growth. Take Hal and Dutchy. His mother's rejection of the baby will push them to go deeper to make hard choices, and to do better in the long run. Challenges evoke our responses, and our responses define us in the moment."

Something inside me goes for a space walk. Certainties and boundaries dissolve. My inner self floats, directionless. For a moment, I leave the mental boat of habit and float freely in the current of unfolding time. I am aware that I can choose to leave my boat and swim, or to board another. But I cannot swim for long.

I lock his gaze and feel the joy of his confidence. "You remind me of Reggie. You have extraordinary faith in life that has nothing to do with belief, ego, or expectations. And you include more than Jews in your 'us.'"

"If a religion excluded anyone, like you for example, I couldn't be a part of it."

I feel almost breathless. "Nor could I. I wouldn't want to participate in any process that would divide me from the divine, or from someone like you."

"Like me?"

"Exactly like you."

Randall raises an eyebrow. I look away. Jos stirs. I begin to sing again. Sometime later, when the baby is dozing, I open my eyes and see that Randall is listening intently, and realize that I am singing the final, pensive verse of the English version of Eileen Aroon. "Youth will in time decay, Eileen Aroon, beauty must fade away, Eileen Aroon, castles are sacked in war, chieftains are scattered far, truth is a fixed star, Eileen Aroon."

Randall stands. He goes to the changing table opposite the crib and pulls a handful of wet wipes from a yellow plastic box. He carries them like an Olympic torch and kneels in front of me to reach over the baby and stroke them along my cheek. As he continues, I realize that he is removing the makeup from my skin. His gestures flow so naturally from the intimacy of the day that I close my eyes and take easy pleasure in his touch. When he comes to my eyes and lips, he brushes them with exquisite tenderness.

When I open my eyes again, he whispers, "I knew you were beautiful."

The moment has arrived when yearning and possibility narrow into a clear question. I am free, for one more moment, to pretend that I don't recognize it, and to allow this moment to pass away. I don't. I take his hand, kiss it, and put it on my chest beside the sleeping baby. "No one's ever said that to me before."

"Maybe they never saw you. Today you showed me the beauty in your heart. It's like a bud about to blossom. I'd like to be there when it opens."

A seed of love sprouts in my heart, sends tendrils into my veins, and penetrates the marrow of my bones. There is no putting the sprout back in the seed. I am surprised to find that I feel no fear or hesitation, only the necessity of loving him without limits. I read in the expression on Randall's lips that he has expected this. I steel myself and look into his eyes again, knowing that I will not be able to conceal my desire, or my vulnerability. When his eyes enter mine, his spirit penetrates my being and leaves an ineffable imprint like a seal in wax. *This must be what it's like to fall in love with a priest! This is what my cousin Paul feared, and may never feel.*

"I bet women fall in love with you all the time," I say.

"They fall in lust. It's not the same. Not the same at all."

Hal and Dutchy appear in the doorway. Their smiles give way to smirks. I stand and put the baby gently on his stomach on the soft white knit sheet of his crib and walk out through the narrow hall, the tidy dining room, and the white living room. At the door, Randall joins me, and we face Hal and Dutchy.

"So, rabbi doctor, you gave Collo a free exam, did you?"

"You have to forgive Hal," Dutchy interjects. "He iss no romantic. Maybe Randall can tell him where to find the heart."

"Thank you for having us," I say.

"We appreciate it." Randall smiles broadly as he shakes Hal's hand.

"Thank you for helping with Jos," Dutchy says. "I'll have to sing to him in Dutch!"

We leave together as in a dream, and the sexual centers that have been filling for days overflow into the space around us. I release my celibacy and my fear. My body becomes his, and his becomes mine. There will be no confining our desire now, no putting it back into manageable forms. It has charged our electric, porous skins, which will merge when we touch, and meld eternally whether or not our bodies join at their roots.

6

Union

When we arrive at Flinders Station and wend our way between incongruous groupings within the scattered night crowd, we brush against ostentatiously dressed patrons of the Arts Center, families returning from a performance of Circus Oz at Town Hall, and young and not-so-young black-clad dancers going to distant nightclubs. When we find a place on the platform, Randall removes his yarmulke, folds it carefully and slips it into his pocket. I am not thinking now; I am in a state of drunken giddiness that entertains an irresistible desire to flirt, to tease, and to play. But first we must wait. We are too distant from our goal to give in to impulse, and so cannot choose but to observe our experience, to consult our intentions, and to make clear choices.

A train rolls into the station. The doors slide open. Inside, old plaid seats marked by cigarette burns and stains exude a clinging sour smell. Across the aisle a few rows down, a suit-clad commuter is dozing. Several rows beyond, a few young men are arguing about whether the Bulldogs will outplay Essendon in the next footy season. Randall and I sit side-by-side on the south side of the train beside curtains that reveal a dark wall. When the passengers have settled, the glaringly lit car is half-full.

As the train pulls out, I put my lips to his ear and whisper, "Let's be consorts for the night. Let's make love."

Randall hesitates. He asks sharply, "Why didn't you have children?"

"Why ask that now?"

"If we get lost in romance or pleasure, the bubble will pop. We'll take away nothing but regret." Randall sucks in air between his teeth. He takes my head gently in his hands and presses his lips between my brows. And then his breath brushes my neck, and he says, "We're going to meet obstacles at every level. If we don't face them in real time, they'll overcome us."

I meet his gaze. The light of his eyes, which is intense from vocation and meditation, is also interrupted by the play of shadows. One minute his heart radiates kind confidence through his gaze, the next his eyes bore into mine with desire, and the next his gaze clouds with vanity, scheming, or doubt. The soul that sustains this play is host to a never-ending soap opera, to a boom and bust mining town on a frontier, to an eternal saga of defiant resistance, to a constant *coup d'etat*. And yet generosity glints like a well-tied fishing fly pinned to the darkness. He is dangerous; he is wonderful.

"My ex-wife says I'm selfish, arrogant, and controlling. I think the same of her. I hated her. I HATED her!" His charisma and good looks are gone. He is a wrathful Tibetan deity with fangs and claws.

"Are you trying to frighten me?" I laugh darkly.

"Why didn't you have children?"

"Wait! If we're going to purify ourselves, I need to prepare. Let me do a few cycles of giving and taking mounted on the breath!"

His wrath is tamed by curiosity. "Of what?"

"I need to do a little *tonglen*, a meditation that purifies negative emotions. Your passion of aversion is more misleading than any bubble of fantasy."

I take a minute to focus my mind, and then breathe in angry sorrow and breathe out love. Soon I am ready to face his demons, and mine. "When I married, I'd spent years bringing up my cousins, so I wasn't in a hurry. And then I didn't want to. I thought I was holding out until we left the farm, but the truth is I that I never wanted him to be the father of my children. And now I want to give birth to a community."

Randall's energy shifts, and I realize that he has committed to a course of action. Together, we have reduced the superabundance of innumerable futures to three possibilities: ecstatic union, disappointment, or both. "Yes, let's practice sacred sex. Together. Tonight. I want to be your consort. But you'll have to guide me."

"We can guide each other."

Our connection grows during the train ride to Ringwood and Lilydale, and continues to grow during the cab ride after. By the time we stand alone in the chilly air at the door of the tasting room in the old white Edwardian house, our fecund bubble of desire has penetrated the ether and joined the winking stars with the resined earth. As my fingers find the flat metal surface of the key, Randall's lips touch the back of my neck. I turn to face him. We are heart to heart and belly-to-belly. His arms enfold me.

Memory takes me back to high school. I am dancing with a boy I hardly know. When the music changes, and we slow dance, his body feels nothing like I imagined, and I am suddenly at home. I had to learn to see him as I felt him. Now, Randall's energy feels higher and denser and narrower than I imagined, and I feel ill at ease, as if his energy body is displaced upward. I whisper, "I didn't expect you to feel like this. It's like we've never met!"

Randall pulls away until our bellies are a foot apart. Then he rests his hands lightly on the curve of my back and says playfully, "Colette's body, this is Randall's. Randall's body, this is Colette's."

To cause our bodies to cohere, I cut and run to the side of the house and turn toward the front lawn. Before disappearing around the corner, I call back over my shoulder, "I want to be chased!"

"Chaste?"

"Run! Come catch me!"

As I run over the smooth, thick turf in the glancing beams of the nightlights, I feel the energy of my flesh spread through my being into my feet. When Randall catches me, his hands reach for my wrist. I take his wrist in my hand and draw him playfully into a spin. When he slows to a dizzy stop, his stiff hair is standing in spikes, he looks like the Greek God Pan with a garland of pine leaves. He staggers slightly. I put my arms around him and pull his belly against mine. His energy feels lower and more open now, and his beating heart is radiating heat. I could hold him like this for hours, drinking in the feel of him.

"There's something I need to ask."

"Feel free."

"You said—" I move to put my palms against his chest, but grip the fabric of his shirtfront instead. "You said you'd been with a lot of women."

"That was a long time ago," he replies glibly. "Now I want one, and only one."

I stiffen. He is avoiding the question, and if I do not object, we will slip into accustomed habits—we will follow our pre-programmed patterns of profane sex.

"What is it?" he asks.

"You were right before. We will face obstacles on every level. One is that I see you banging all those women, and wonder what you were doing, and what it did to you. If you don't face that with me, we'll feed the shadow."

"Let's talk inside, where we can see each other."

"Let's see each other like this." I put my arms around his neck and press my lips to his right ear. We are standing cheek to cheek. "Wasn't it like giving out bits of your soul? Andy wanders the night like a tomcat."

Randall tenses. "How do you know what Andy does at night?"

"This is a small place. Everyone who works here knows that you're staying the night with me."

"They won't know the details," he objects.

"Andy used to sleep with every woman he could. It couldn't have been good for him. He might as well have scattered bits of his soul on the wind."

Randall lifts his arms so that he is holding my back with exquisite tenderness. "I didn't lose. I gained. Nearly every time."

"Wasn't it like taking something? I used to see Andy as a thief in the night, or as an addict who needed help."

Randall says lovingly, "I can't speak for Andy, but when you make love, and don't expect it to be something more than it is, you bring new life into being. It's like a mutual gift, and can even be a gift to the world."

"Is that how it is for you now?"

Randall does not reply. I realized with shock that he has been talking of his love life in the past tense. It seems abominable that Randall, or any man of such gifts, could be impotent in any way. My body would give him physical love tonight, not as a gift, but as a sacrificial offering. My mind has a sole vision, which is to share my being with Randall in a way that mends every kind of brokenness, from the rough moments of the day to the deep wounds of the past, from the carnal to the ethereal. My being opens completely. I feel no barrier now.

He finally replies, "If we stay aware like this, we'll share our best and parry our worst."

We breathe as one. The breeze brings the bark of a distant owl, the rattling of a gum tree's long leaves, the green tea taste of grass, and the tang of Yarra dust. Even as we touch eternal truths, time is passing, and life is changing.

"Ours can be a story of sexual healing."

"For both of us, and more, I hope."

I release his neck and ruffle his shirt. "This is like a book cover, and you're like the *Poetic Edda,* and I'm ready to open it."

He laughs. The sound of it comes into my chest like a Chopin glissando into the heart of Georges Sand. "Let's savor the not knowing, the wondering."

I release him and take his hand in mine. We retrace our steps in the near-darkness. "Does Kabbalah have sacred sexuality?"

"In a way. As we see it, the child's character is formed by the attitudes of the parents at the time of conception. So Jewish men, especially orthodox men, place a high value on making sex pleasurable for women."

I grip his hand. We walk through an invisible but dense barrier created by my teachers, who cast sexual pleasure in the roles of sin and enemy. Beyond this barrier lies the world I entered once before, on a beach at night. For a moment, I am transported to the place of yes where sex is cleansing, nourishing, and leaves a trace of blessing that cannot be blotted out. As we reach the door, a thought forms and lumbers across the vault of my mind.

"Everyone I know but Reggie, and you, treats sex as filthy or naughty. Sacred sex is so taboo that the mere mention of it can unleash dark forces."

"Why do you say that?"

"The secrecy, for one thing."

"Perhaps it's the secrecy that keeps it sacred."

"Or keeps it dirty. That way initiation confers privilege."

I release Randall's hand, put the key in the lock, and turn it. The door swings open with a creak. "Would you like to start with a sip of Botrytis?"

"Let's toast Reggie."

The damp air of the tasting room envelops us in sweet decay. Randall closes and locks the door as I duck behind the counter, grab an open bottle by the neck, and pour samples of amber nectar into two of the glasses that are waiting on the smooth marble.

"What is Botrytis, anyway?"

"It's a dessert wine like port or sherry, but lighter."

Randall sniffs the cloying bouquet and takes a scant sip. His mouth curls into a cagey smile. He reaches across the marble counter, holds my nape in one hand, and darts his tongue over and between my lips, leaving a slippery trace of caramel and a hint of chili chocolate. Then he grabs a strand of my loose long hair, dips it in the wine and sucks it dry. "It's sweet and pungent, like the air in the room."

I down my glass and then walk around the counter to take his arm. His lips catch mine with a playful kiss like the nip of a soft turtle's beak, and then he dances lightly backwards. "Where's the bedroom? We can begin any way we want: sleep, take a bath, look for birthmarks."

I've reached a hidden boundary I can't see. I can only try to walk boldly through it. I grip the neck of the Botrytis bottle in two tense hands, and walk to the stairs and up as if toward a medieval test of valor. At the top of the stairs, I pass the boundary formed by the closed sofa bed and enter the other world of

Reggie's alcove, where I place the bottle on the low altar beside the sheepskins and turn on the lamp.

"I'd like to shower," I say tremulously.

"Are you alright?"

"I didn't realize how intense this would be. It's different than dialogue."

"I hoped it would be intense. It's a sign that we're open, and healing."

"I didn't think of that."

I scurry into the bathroom, wash hastily, and wrap my naked body in a bath sheet. When I emerge, Randall kisses me sweetly on the cheek and goes in to take his turn. I retreat beyond the altar table that holds candles and jars of oil and kneel at the far end of Reggie's thick stack of sheepskins. I close my eyes and meditate on my heart. Free-floating fear and regret bloom into a lily of pain, then pass away. My slumbering equanimity begins to awaken. *Thank you, Reggie, for all that you've taught me.*

I open my eyes to see Randall kneeling opposite me, knees apart, his tailbone suspended between his heels. Sandy hair spreads out on either side of his breastbone like a pair of wings. Wiry pubic hair forms a tangled nest for pink testicle-eggs. His erect, blue-lined penis is pointing at my heart. Color seems to rise from the ground and to infuse the air with earthen tones of amber and ochre.

My eyelids crash like window sashes. "I'm not ready to see your—your—"

"Lingam. Let's use holy words that are neutral to us, like lingam and yoni."

"Okay," I say tensely.

When I am breathing regularly, and my equanimity has revived, I open my eyes and see his kind, radiant joy, which invites us to be like newborns whose pure souls are still joined with the Other. I am at ease enough to regard his body without fear. I notice that there is no white shadow where a swimsuit would have blocked the sun. "You're not tan!"

He frowns and sets his arms over his pelvis, cupping his hands over his penis. "Unusual for Australia."

"I didn't know that Jews were dark."

"Jews aren't dark," he blurts irritably.

"Have you been—is it the nude beaches?" I ask shyly.

Randall's frown eases. One corner of his mouth lifts in a smile. "Nude bathing is a great pleasure."

"I don't think I'd like it. Not yet. I'm sorry about what I said about Jews being dark. It's just that you're the same shade as my grandmother, and I thought for a minute that it was natural."

His expression shifts to reveal astonishment and then that hawk-like look. "Your grandmother?"

I blanch. I've never discussed my grandmother's color with anyone but my grandparents and my mother and brother. I begin slowly. "My grandmother didn't talk about her background. It was her secret, a family secret. When we asked, she would say that she didn't know. That made us curious, and apprehensive. When she died Sean got my mother to tell us everything she knew, which was that Grandma spoke Algonquin and came from near Lac-Rapide. A lot of First Nations people live there. When Grandpa met her in Montreal, he married her and took her to live in an Acadian community in Rhode Island. My mom lived there until she moved to Peoria with my dad."

"Was your grandmother taken from her family?"

"She might have been. But she was so ashamed of her roots that I think she might have had another secret. Her mother might have been, um, well, sexually assaulted. Grandma was light, really light. She could pass, and she did."

"Maybe she was a love child."

"You mean a bastard."

"I mean her parents might have made love and then been separated."

"It's a thought. My brother and I go around and around about it. But it's no use. We don't even know her real name. Sean thinks of her as Métis, but the identity politics of that are complicated. Plus Métis tend to see the Québécois as different, which may be fair."

He studies my face. "I don't see any signs of indigenous blood in you."

I sigh. "You can see her face in my cheekbones." I touch my fingertips to them as if to feel my blood. "Sean and I grew up surrounded by Scandinavians with similar bone structure, so no one noticed, not even Melissa."

He seems troubled. "I didn't expect this."

"Is it—is it a problem? Grandma was Catholic, too."

He shakes his head and then laughs tenderly. "Not a problem; a mystery, maybe. I don't know much about Indians. Not the ones here—there, I mean."

I smile. "It's good to surprise you. You always surprise me. Seeing anything through your eyes is like seeing it for the first time."

I look at the space between our hearts and see a vision of our lineages flowing together. They form complex currents of awareness and flesh; eddies of perception, sensation, and understanding; and confluences of energy and interbeing. We are already becoming one soul. It is too late to undo the rash choice that brought us here together tonight, stripped of clothing and of voluntary barriers to union.

Randall and I sit facing each other at the threshold of the created and uncreated worlds. We are ready, almost, to join our lives through our bodies. I gasp at the recognition that our bodily joining will, indeed, be full and holy. Unholy obstacles still divide us, though, as in this moment, when I seem to see Steven's eyes looking into mine with lewd contempt. My breath catches deep in my chest.

"Steven always—"

"Wait! Tell me about your experience, not his. Let's keep this between us."

"Good! But can we turn off the lights? This is hard."

Randall's face radiates concern. As I close my eyes again, and try to regain my calm, I hear him arranging items on the table and fumbling with matches and switches. When I open my eyes he is sitting on his haunches with a towel around his waist. Two small votive candles illuminate the room just enough for us to see into each other's eyes.

"Better?" he asks tenderly.

"Much!" And then, without thought, I dive for his chest and throw my arms around his neck.

I freeze.

My mind goes blank.

My gut contracts.

My breath catches in my throat.

I clench my hands and manage to utter, "I'm afraid."

"I know," he whispers breathlessly. "It's all right. I know how to hold you."

I cling to him like a toddler to an elder's leg, grateful for his mass and warmth. I release my jaw and choke out, "I don't deserve your kindness." When I hear my words mortification moves me deeper into the curse of shame.

Randall says gently, "You've steadied me tonight; now let me steady you. Think of what Catholics say—the closer you get to God, the greater the inner resistance."

I begin to sob. I am a child confined by frightening rules. "It's not that. It's that I'm not good enough. I'm not. If I touch the sacred, I'll only defile it."

"You have to let go of those thoughts. They lead nowhere."

I nod. I try to pry fear's fingers away from the jugular vein of reason. Reggie talks about letting go. The books I've read all talk of it. I've said it, too, but I haven't understood it. I turn it into a mantra. *Let go... let go... let go.*

"That's right. Take some deep breaths."

"It's easy to say let go, and to imagine doing it, but how?"

"Lean on me, now, and let it happen."

I move to rest my head on his shoulder, but stop and grip his nape. "I—I trust the sacred in you. I do."

"And I trust the holy sparks that we will touch together, and redeem."

I take a deep sigh, but am not ready to release him.

"Give me that gift?" he asks gently. "Trust me to give you pleasure?"

"I don't know what that means. You may, but I don't. I don't."

"It's as you said earlier, it's up to us."

Gradually, I release him and sit back on my heels. Air rushes into his throat. I squeezed the breath out of him. "I'm sorry."

Randall mock-strangles himself and falls playfully to the side. I can't help but laugh. He is funny. He is the rabbi comedian who knows how to break out of hell with comedy. When his humor has freed me, he springs up and winks. "Just release it. Let everything go."

I feel him do it. I nod and take a deep breath. My awareness begins to re-expand. I become aware of the whirr of the refrigerator, and of the sputtering of a votive.

"Look at me," he says softly.

I realize that I have been staring at his chest. I raise my gaze to his hesitantly, and see that his gaze is gentle, loving, and strong. In moments, it overwhelms me with a power I can't hold. I snap shut my eyes and shake my head. "It's too much!"

"My desire is strong."

"You mean complicated?"

He laughs a sharp outbreath. "It's pretty simple right now. Just let me know what you want, and when you want it, and you'll find me ready."

I inch toward him and place my palms gingerly on the hair wings of his chest. Warmth enters, but he has stilled his energy, and is balancing on a tightrope between eagerness and patience. His desire does not overwhelm me. I slide my palms up to his nape, and then up to the bony back of his skull, and raise my eyes to his. They hold me steady through the thrill of this first nearly-naked touch. I ease my towel-covered breasts into the fold between his chest and belly.

His lips curl back, exposing glistening teeth and tongue. "Go easy! This is going to be harder than I thought. Let me try something?"

He pulls back, takes my hand in his, and places my palm on his breastbone. He puts his on mine. His body opens in welcome. I feel room upon room opening as if each is waiting for me to enter. When we are looking easily and lovingly into each other's eyes, he inches closer and rests his palms lightly on either side of my sacrum. Arousal fills the space between my legs. My breath comes quickly. As I breathe, the energy spreads and the arousal eases. We wait. I move my belly toward his. I stop abruptly when

I feel his hard erection. My body tenses with arousal. My breath sends the arousal outward to fill the shared cup of our being. My panic passes. He moves closer, and we fill with another wave of arousal and awareness.

You'd think I'd never done this before.

You haven't. Not with him.

Not with a man as aware and as loving as he is.

He is blessing me, and I open to bless him. As we share this, we live into blessing and begin to become it.

Randall whispers, "Tell me about your night on the beach."

I think back and remember my back opening to the earth. "I was in heaven. It was easy, and loving."

"Can you feel that now?"

I picture Randall as I saw Andy then, hovering over me, eyes filled with urgent demands. "This is better, but this time it isn't me with the sacred, it's me with you."

"And through me, the sacred." Randall's forehead eases slowly toward mine. I tense; he waits. We repeat this until his forehead is touching mine, and his breath is stirring the hairs on my lip. Our energy expands and unites above our crowns; our state of arousal eases. When he has caressed my forehead with his for a full minute, I gasp. "This is wonderful, this kissing without lips. I had no idea."

"Let's talk of wonder. I feel it when I look at you, so perfect and mysterious, like a miracle."

I am overwhelmed for a time, after which I say, "I feel your wonder, and your strength, and more than us, through us."

Randall smiles mischievously, "And no celibacy in the mix."

I laugh lightly and say, "Let's improvise an invocation. Something that invites the sacred, and expresses our intention."

"I can't sustain that level of awareness and think at the same time." Randall laughs a single outbreath, tosses his thick head of hair, and takes a deep breath. "This night, I offer to you my *nefesh*, *ruach*, and *neshama*, and what is mine of the higher levels of my soul. May our sparks reunite, and so help to bring the universal soul nearer to the Garden."

Overwhelmed, I close my eyes. When I open them again, I gaze into his and say, "I offer you my physical body, energy body, and spiritual body on this sacrificial altar. May we unite and become whole, and fill each other to overflowing, and offer that overflow to the eternal."

He says, "When we come together, may we recognize that we are always in heaven, and realize that heaven as we unite in the flesh."

"Make me a promise," I say boldly. "Any promise you can keep."

After what seems like many minutes, he says, "I will do what I am able to co-create whatever it is that we are meant to bring forth together."

I release him and go to the table to pour more wine into our glasses. When the wine overflows onto the tray, I stop and say, "Like those who tend the vines, pick the grapes, and make this wine, I will tend to you, and fill the cup of your body with loving pleasure until our hearts open."

Randall tenses slightly. "Those are big promises! Better to say too little."

"We can start over, if you like."

I put down my glass and take up his embrace, moving my lips slowly toward his. He accepts my lips and responds just enough to invite my mouth to explore his. Slowly, so slowly that it seems we are not moving at all, I feel our mouths forming a shared language of touch that is tied to being.

The rest of our bodies join in this creation. The taste of him arouses my skin like the taste of the best wine; it molds my energy to his; it plays on my heartstrings until they resonate with his; and when my tongue touches his with exquisite delicacy, our whole bodies listen, conform, wait, search, take delight, and begin again.

After a time, my yoni opens like the dewy petals of a sun-kissed flower, and I say, "On the beach, I felt adoration, and ecstasy. It was like making love with saints, and with Solomon and all his wives, and their spiritual descendants."

"The wives were allegorical."

"What do you mean?"

"The story is about knowing the covenant intimately, so much that you seem to have shared a marriage bed with it, and with everyone else who has known and loved it."

"I don't see a difference. Perhaps if I understood his Song."

"I'll tell you. Tonight you'll make love to me, and to the covenant through me, but you won't know it directly unless you choose to love it as I do."

I try to think, and then I let the words come. "I choose to know the sacred in both of us with the tender care of prayer, and in sight of the objects that Reggie chose as images of the divine."

"*Amein.*"

I pull back and pull my towel away. I hear Randall breathing deeply and quickly, and feel the space between us thicken and shrink. We continue breathing deeply together until it expands. I spread my knees. Randall drops his towel. His dusky lingam pulses with his heart. His eyes radiate desire under close control. We breathe again, allowing our bodies to fill, and to overflow. Very slowly, Randall embraces me, and tightens his embrace until my breasts are pressed inside the fold of his chest. Then he caresses my mouth with his lips and tongue, seeking and finding the places where our energies flow together. It is the first kiss of union, through which our two bodies become one.

Soon, I become impatient. I pull away, lie back on the soft skins, and say eagerly, "Come into me, now. Come inside my skin!"

Randall smiles sweetly and asks, "Turn face down?"

I take time to breathe deeply, and then turn to rest my belly on the soft white wool. I have no idea what to expect, but my trust is absolute, now, and I feel only anticipation when his knees straddle my waist, and a glass bottle clinks, and fragrances of sandalwood and frankincense infuse the air.

After a pause pregnant with anticipation, Randall's warm hands stroke the skin of my back, filling my flesh with the scintillating light of his being. When the light of his life has enveloped my body, his fingertips play a romantic cadenza on the insturment of my arousal, and the nearness of his phallus awakens my sexual centers. As he caresses my back with his mouth and tongue, the boundaries of our shared awareness expand, and we experience our soul union like a first taste of chocolate, a first whiff of lilac, or a first orgasm. After some time, when it seems that we have become one with all that lies above and below, his weight shifts, his chest slips slowly up my back, and the tip of his lingam glides between my legs. I feel a first sweet shock of intimate touch. My yoni swells painfully and overflows. A wave of liquid sunlight flows up my back.

Randall moans a long, slow wave of shared ecstasy.

A resonant laugh penetrates my back.

"A valley!"

"Sit up?" he asks.

Randall guides me. I sit facing him with my legs wrapped around him. His lingam presses my belly. I realize with delight that we are sitting as tantrikas do.

"Look into my eyes."

I lock his gaze and feel union. I gasp. "But we're only touching."

Randall's lips turn up.

I whisper, "Bring your awareness to the place below your navel. Hindus visualize Brahma. Try to see light, or a flame."

"Wait! Let's just gaze for now."

We sit in stillness. Our concentration deepens. Boundaries dissolve. Inner and outer flow together. A part of my mind is amazed that though we have known each other for only a week, we are profoundly and irrevocably connected. Abruptly, a bright white light in my chest pulls my head backward, breaking our gaze. I let the light take me. Many minutes later, when it dims, and my head eases forward, Randall is smiling. I lock his gaze again and say, "A yoga *kriya*! My heart opened."

He smiles with a touch of triumph. "It began to open."

Randall motions me to lie back on the thick, soft wool, which smells of him, and of oil, and of the fluids of my yoni. He straddles me again and pleasures my front as he pleasured my back. This time I watch him, and marvel at his mastery of our energy. When he reaches mischievously between my legs to touch the wet mouth of my yoni, and to initiate another low, long valley, I look into his eyes, breathe, and hold the energy of his gaze. When it doesn't stop, I whisper, "You, you!"

"You sure?" He is losing the will to hold back from the cascade of release.

"Yes!"

"Take it easy." Randall lies on his belly, one leg bent to accommodate his erection. "I'm close."

"You can release whenever you like."

He shakes his head. "Inside, together."

I pour a dram of oil in my palm, spread it over my hands, and stroke his back. I am not as skilled. Our arousal ebbs. I close my eyes and seek out his energy, and then caress him shyly with my fingers and lips, ending with a long sucking kiss that begins between the dimples of his sacrum and ends at his hairline. He moans as my pendant breasts and hair move up his back and my body comes to rest on his. His moan becomes a groan; my juices pool on the back of his thigh.

"Come inside me now?"

He nods, turns, and motions me to lie on my back. He lowers his body over mine and kisses me deeply, and then rises to his knees and pulls my calves over his shoulders. He pushes inside me gently, slowly, and deeply. Our gazes lock as our roots meet. His being fills mine. I envision the place of our joining as the white yin of my yoni and its clitoral dot of black yan becoming one with the black yan of his lingam and the white yin dot behind them.

I feel as a long, low valley of earthy, fertile yin. "Did you feel that?"

He laughs with the outbreath.

"Did you know that my ecstasy would be a valley?"

Confusion muddles his concentration. "There's no one ecstasy."

"If you shared mine, will I share yours?"

"Let's find out."

He glides in and out, deeply and shallowly, slowly and quickly., a series of patterns that begins with seven slow and shallow followed by two fast and deep, and shifting gradually toward faster and deeper. I see nothing but his eyes. I feel the sheet, the bead of sweat in my scalp, the touch of his thigh hair, but none of it breaks our connection, or raises a boundary between his pleasure and mine. At intervals he stops, panting, and we carry energy through our bodies on the breath. We ride wave after wave of yin, eyes locked. After a time, he begins to turn my body slowly, like a potter leaving his imprint on the encircling wall of my full yoni. My vision of our joining pulsates as it turns. When his mastery of all that we are is complete, he pauses like a painter who holds back before adding one brushstroke too many and then gives himself up to climax. I feel his peak as my own. When the last wave of ecstasy breaks, he falls beside me on his back.

After a time he whispers, "Someday I'll be able to peak without coming."

I smile. I feel no lack, and have no desire to imagine more. "When you're inside me, every moment is timeless."

After a longer interval, he whispers, "We should say a prayer or a blessing."

"Yes! Let's dedicate our practice, like Buddhists, to all living beings."

After our dedication, Randall turns me away and lies behind me, his body nestling mine. When we are both drifting between wakefulness and sleep, I laugh deeply. "That was the first time anyone's ever made love to my whole being."

"That was the first time I've made love with someone who wasn't lost in a fantasy. Which means—" Randall turns me on my back and looks into my eyes intently. "There's something I have to tell you. It matters to me, and might matter to you."

"What is it?"

"I'm not what you think."

"You're from Mars?"

"I'm being serious."

"I think you're the man who just made love to me, and let me make love to him. I can't imagine anything that could come between us now."

"You may not—well, I'll tell you then. I wasn't born to my parents. I was adopted."

"Ah. Why would that matter?"

"I'm Jewish by their choice and mine, not by blood."

"That's beautiful. Coercion is a terrible basis for faith. Why are you trembling? Are you afraid of Jewish law?"

"That's part of it," he replies. His forehead is drawn into a crease that is like a curtain suspended above his face. His gaze is resting on my chin. He is afraid to tell me, afraid of being judged.

"I can't imagine anyone judging you for the circumstances of your birth, which were obviously beyond your control. We have to accept our beginnings as they are, even when we don't know what they are."

He takes a deep sigh and looks fiercely into my eyes. "Ten percent of paternity is misreported."

"I don't understand."

"One in ten Americans is mistaken in the identity of their biological father."

"Are you saying that one in ten mothers lied?"

"No. Some fathers know and choose to keep it to themselves."

"So Grandma wasn't so unusual."

"It's different in Utah, where only one in a hundred fathers is misreported."

"Were you born a Mormon?"

"No. I was born to a Muslim father and a Hindu mother."

"Ah. I can see how that might distress your Jewish friends."

"It isn't that. You—you noticed my accent. It's the R. It comes out when I'm tired, or distracted."

I rack my memory. "You were born in India? That's unusual for someone our age, isn't it? People adopted locally back then."

"It wasn't an ordinary adoption. My parents didn't give me

up. They—um—they died."

"How awful! I'm sorry. How old were you?"

"Five."

"How bereft you must have felt! How wonderful that a good family took you in."

"There's more. It's—I—um, they, um."

I realize then that he is afraid to remember, afraid of judging himself. I put my hand over his heart. "Take your time."

He closes his eyes and breathes deeply. "My family—birth family—was caught in a religious conflict."

"Between Muslims and Hindus?"

Randall nods. "My mother married against her family's wishes. Things are different there. It was as if an antebellum Southern belle married a black man. They—the clans—took revenge. They, uh, they—they."

I want to absorb my shock and sorrow and his, but the space between us is too open, and my system cannot contain his feelings. Tears well up, run across the bridge of my nose, and drop onto the pillow.

He wipes my tears with his thumb. "I wasn't home. I had gone to the riverbank with the son of a visiting doctor. We went to play. When we came up to the road we saw his father's car. It stopped and we climbed in and he drove away. He didn't stop for hours. He drove all the way to his house in Bombay. There he told me what had happened. I didn't believe him for a while."

"How long did you stay with him?"

"I don't remember. I remember climbing into the lap of my American father, and flying across the ocean. I remember that he and my mother moved to France, then to California so that they could conceal the adoption. It was such a complete break that I lost all of my early memories. Until I went back to visit the, um, the site."

"Randall, I think I must be missing something. Why would that matter to me, except in that it still upsets you? Is there something else you haven't told me?"

"When you spoke of your grandmother, I could feel that it was hard for you to release the secret. It's been the same for me. Only my brother and parents know. I never told my wife. I haven't reconciled with it."

"Does it give you too many choices, make you wonder if you're Hindu, Muslim, or Jewish?"

"I'm Jewish. That much I know. And I'm more, too, and glad of it. It's the violence I can't reconcile. I was born into a family of lovers and murderers."

"Your own personal Holocaust—and you've felt that you had to handle it all on your own."

"And ... and to know that we all have the potential to go that way, whether we admit it or not."

"You've been a lover and dedicated your life to bringing new life into the world."

Randall sighs and opens his eyes. His gaze is fierce. "I've tried all my life to be a lover of life. But the other creeps in. There's violence in surgery. It's well intended, but bloody and sometimes savage. Every time I make the incision I notice the violence."

"You chose life. You chose right."

"I'm choosing now. With you, here, in this place, I see a way to choose love with all my heart and all my being and all my body. The consort path is the way to turn destruction into creation. I want to commit to it."

I take his right palm and put it over my heart, and then put my hand over his. I kiss his forehead and whisper, "*D'accord, mon amour, d'accord.* I will go with you when you go home."

7

Experiment

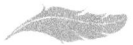

Trailing a cloud of steam, I pull up my towel and scurry out of the bathroom of Randall's Chicago condo. I pass through the sky-lit foyer and the relentlessly male slate-floored living room—with its chrome and black leather furnishings—into the carpeted, rosewood-perfumed refuge of my brightly colored chamber. I close the door, drop the towel, and leap between the glossy red sheets to lie on the soft pillows and wait for Randall's long-delayed embrace.

Let today be the day when we practice sacred sex again, and talk about what we will bring into the world, about our beloved third.

My time in bed is like all the rest of my time in Chicago: dreamlike, slow, indefinite. When I arrived, the noise and rush of the airport made it seem as if Randall were more alive when he met me with a passionate embrace and drove me to this condominium in Printer's Row. His suggestive talk of teaching me to sing the Song of Songs with him thrilled me, but I soon saw that what I had taken for bright new clarity was stress-driven haphazard hurry. Even before we'd brought in my bags, he took me to the dining table and pulled me down on it to couple and climax explosively.

We spent the next few weeks furnishing a chamber for consort practice. It was easy for him to follow the simple rituals of shopping for a bed, and sheets, and the items that we would put on our bedside altar to remind us of our purpose. We bounced on mattresses, tried meditation cushions, and bought everything we needed, and more, we painted the walls, hung the curtains, and made the myriad of tiny decisions that readied the room for our use.

The room looked perfect. It is easy for Randall to seek perfection, and it was—and is still—easy for me to believe that he is lying fallow for the moment—that when he has caught up at work, and finished with the custody battle, he will have the energy to explore the artistry of transformative partnership. He is confident that we will soon think and act with one mind and the resources of more than two. He will give up his old life then, he says, and we will turn our loving attention to the shared life we intend to build, discovering how best to seed the intangible realm of the uncreated.

And so, with anticipation, I say every day, "Let's unite tonight," and every morning he smiles a sly promise, fondles my breasts, and leaves for work. When he calls to say that he is on his way home, I pluck, shower, shampoo, and oil my body and go to our chamber to wait. He arrives late, slumps on the squeaky leather sofa, and waits to be waited on—or, if especially tense, leads me to the couch to couple quickly before sleep.

I stare at the ceiling now and say aloud, "Story Time. I have no story."

Like Randall, I have lost the thread of my life. I am a fish in a terrarium, a chintz sofa in a modernist space, a holographic twist of yin embedded in a plastic male ego. I am out of place in this anonymous condo, this plywood and sheetrock testament to transience in housing, and, increasingly, in my own skin.

Let today be the day when our lives begin to make sense.

I stand and stretch my arms to the ceiling, put on a robe and slippers, and scuff out to the foyer to call my brother and tell him about my visit to Peoria to see Maman. I want him to envision her sitting on the sofa in a housedress, clutching a rosary to her bony chest with blue-veined hands. I want him to know that the wall paint behind her is peeling, and that the house smells of neglect. I want him to come with me next time, so that we can tend to her and to her house.

"Hey there, *mon frère.*"

"Ha, *ma soeur.* Where are you?"

"I'm living in sin with a Jew in Chicago!" I reply provocatively.

Sean gasps. My coarse-mouthed, tavern-tough musician brother is shocked by my situation. "Hoo-wee. *Ma soeur* in synagogue!"

"Our plan is to meditate together in the bedroom."

"I'm not touching that one."

"Ta gueule."

The receiver at his end of the line clatters. "Put that down!" he shouts, presumably castigating one of his sons. After an ear-deafening crackle, he comes back on to say, "What are you doing? You were just getting into the wine business and now—Hey!" he shouts again. "Break that bow and you're eatin' it for dinner!" He sighs heavily. "Ciao for now, *ma soeur.* Call me when you get your shit together." The line goes dead.

I hold on to the phone as if afraid that it, too, may abandon me. My brother is too busy to speak to me. Everyone is too busy to speak to me.

I return to my chamber, sit on the *zafu* cushion in front of our small altar, and look for inspiration. I look to the framed leaf of Hebrew writing, the small iron lingam topped with dried rose petals, the icon of Mary, and the serene figurine of the Buddha.

I light the smoky incense that takes me outside of time, reminding me of the pecan wood drawer where Grandfather stored his tobacco. And then I realize what I need: I pull a photo of Reggie from the drawer.

"If you were in my place, would you leave?" I ask. "You put up with a lot to be with your consort. Should I?"

Reggie smiles unperturbed. I light a votive candle in a lotus-shaped glass and invite it to stand in for the light of her wisdom.

"I'm not getting on without you, Reg."

I reckon you and Randall should support each other's practices.

"Oh, Reg, he won't practice! And the worst thing is that it may be because I'm not Jewish. He says it isn't, but he denies all the hard stuff now."

I tried to warn you.

"I know you did. But there's some potential between us that's bigger than both of us, and that we haven't yet brought into being."

The bubble's bound to burst. Romantic love's a delusion.

"It's more than romance. It's our third. When we fall asleep, or sit quietly, I feel an unborn presence, a purpose and project we have yet to create."

If you want a baby, you should try now, shouldn't you, before your time runs out.

"Maybe that's what he wants. But right now this is only an affair."

You're a concubine, then, are you?

My heart aches. "Yes, I'm a kept woman, a pox doctor's tart. And given that Randall is his job, I'm not even kept by a man. I'm kept by a job."

You wanted insight, didn't you?

"I didn't come here to go it alone. I miss community. I can barely stand to visit some of the restaurants that buy your wine. I can't tune out the violence, or greed, or poverty, or hatred, or homelessness. I see all the hard truths, now, and little reason for hope."

You need more than wisdom and compassion. Don't forget strength.

"I must have been taking strength from you, because I don't feel any here."

Randall is taking it. Are you coming back now?

"No. Not now. Not yet."

Try working with the energy body. It'll strengthen your practice.

"I will."

The phone rings like a bell signaling the end of this discussion. Eager for any distraction from my sexual tension, I jump up and run into the foyer to answer.

"Colette?"

"Melissa!"

"Sorry it took me so long to call. We were out of town. It's been crazy. I might get paged any minute, but I didn't want to put it off any longer!"

"I'm glad. I'm only a thousand miles away now. We should chat more often."

"And you have so much news! I have to say that I thought Randall might make a pass, but I never thought he'd bring you home!"

"Thanks."

"I don't mean it that way. It's that Randall's always had a clear agenda for himself, and I can't see how you fit into it."

"We do have a shared purpose."

"I knew it! What is it?"

"We wanted to pursue some of the things we learned from Reggie."

"You're going to make wine?"

"It's hard to explain." I hesitate. Melissa doesn't suffer fools gladly. After skipping a few beats, I say, "Okay. I may as well tell you. You're a big girl now. The truth is we intended to be consorts and practice tantric sex."

"You had tantric sex with Reggie?"

"No! But we learned a lot from her. And I'm really missing her. I always felt great around her and now every day is a struggle."

"Maybe you have feelings for her that you haven't acknowledged."

I can see the frown on Melissa's face and feel the prick of her thorny opinions. I do the tantric trick of seeing us as if from a distance, and realize that she is struggling with her own difficulties. I laugh and say easily, "Goodness! You sound like Steve."

"Well, when different people say the same thing…"

"It isn't that. Reggie exudes happiness, and when I'm near her I get to soak it up, and feel happier than I can feel on my own."

After a long pause, Melissa says, "Okay, I can see that. You've always done that for me."

"Well, thanks for saying that. And how are you? Randall tells me you've had a rough time with Dan. I'm sorry I haven't been a better friend."

There is an uncomfortable silence. I suppress the reflex to twist the cord of the Princess phone I used when we were teens. Finally, she replies tensely, "Things are evening out. Sometime when you and I have a few days together, I'll tell you the whole saga. Right now I'm concerned about you."

"To be perfectly honest, things aren't going at all well. All my energy pours into Randall, and from Randall into his job. I can't keep up."

"Give the man a break. He's got a big job. You have no idea."

"I wish that were true. The most disturbing thing about his workaholism is that he can create a beautiful calm when he's doing something intense, but he can't relax in the downtime the way he did down under. He amuses himself by watching shockingly violent films that sustain his tension. And he—well, I've found some prescriptions here that seem unnecessary, and I'm not sure what to do about it."

"I wouldn't worry. Randall knows how to take care of himself, unlike some of our colleagues who have crashed and burned. If you want to be with him, you may have to accept that his job takes a big toll."

"On both of us. I don't remember applying for his job, or accepting it."

"He has a lot of responsibility on his shoulders, and the custody battle must be cranking it up big time."

"Too true. He can't even talk about it. I could handle it if we were practicing tantra. But we're not."

"That sounds pretty calculating."

"It's realistic. He's painted me into a corner, Lissy, the same way Steve did. We're turning me into the enabler of his workaholism, at the cost of our shared happiness. I'm going to have to find a compelling reason to stay, or get a bright idea about how to cope. Or leave."

"Maybe you'll find it easier when you have place of your own and you're more independent."

"I didn't come here to be independent, I came here to be interdependent. If it doesn't work out, I'll go back and pick up where I left off."

"Left off what? Getting into the wine industry?"

I take a deep breath and plunge in. "Remember when we agreed that I should tell you what was going on with me, and that you should listen?"

"Yes."

"Are you ready to try it?"

"My goodness, what did I just miss?"

"Tantric sex isn't just sex. It's a spiritual practice. It's a way of life. I've been doing inner work, a kind of cross between modern psychology and ancient Buddhist and Hindu practice. Randall was doing similar work through Kabbalah. That's what I came here for, that's what he's avoiding, and that's what I'm determined to do. I love Randall. We're one body now. But I won't be ruled by his subconscious mind."

"Can't you do whatever it is by yourself until after the custody decision?"

"Up to a point. Randall's need for control is coopting my energy and wearing me down."

"I worry about you going back. Reggie sounds like a cultist. It's scary."

"You really don't understand. It's about me controlling my own mind. Not Reggie. Not Randall. Me. Reggie knows how to create and to share a joyful, peaceful state of mind, and when I'm around her I can do it, too. With Randall working against me, I can't."

"Are you sure it's a good idea?"

"Absolutely. I see the results already. I had a good talk with Steve last week."

"That could be construed as positive."

"It is positive. Absolutely. Not to mention hard and utterly amazing."

"Maybe you're just feeling let down. The biochemical rush of falling in love was bound to wear off. And life in Australia might have been exciting, but that was bound to become routine too."

"You need to understand how lonely I am here. Chicago feels like a city with a million closed doors. I could end up frozen out, like I was in Maine."

"But routine is normal," Melissa insists. "We couldn't walk if we had to think about how to take each step."

"Routine can be wonderful, but it needn't be burdensome, or depressing. I may need to leave to create a routine I can sustain."

"I hope things work out. Speaking of which, if you see John, tell him—" Melissa's voice cracks. I can visualize a knot of determination forming in her chin. "Tell him that I'm thinking of him, and will think of him. Always."

"Sure. Sure thing."

A beeper sounds in the background. "I have to go. Look out for yourself. Randall's broken a lot of hearts. I'm lucky I only loved him a little."

She hangs up. My heart hurts with the recognition that Melissa is worried because she understands how I will feel if I were to leave Randall. I realize that our old patterns of mutual irritation conceal a deep bond that is near to the kind I am missing. I go to the meditation cushion to gather my wits, and enter quickly into deep absorption that ends only when I hear Randall's voice; only after do I realize that I have spent time beyond the bounds of awareness.

I open my eyes to see his fine form leaning stagily against the doorframe. I can tell now when he is posing, when he is aware that someone is looking at him. He is vain and also tense and determined to seem relaxed. I close my eyes again to avoid the pretense of his stance, which is a reminder of the false promises he made, few but treasured and therefore missed all the more.

"Put on that dress I bought you! We have reservations at Le Jardin! Everyone's talking about it!" Randall smiles a knockoff of *joie de vivre*. There is an undertone of aggression in his voice. He is going to insist that we relax and have fun, and will expect us to appear to do so.

"We were going to make love. I was going to cook for you."

I look to assess his reaction, but Randall has disappeared. I hear the shower pound the tub, and then hear the bathmat lift like a page tearing from a wall calendar. I go to the chamber alone and put on the clingy red dress and high heels that he likes, in which I feel a high-rent escort, and add the fancy opal earrings that he gave me back when he was eager to woo me. I brush out my hair and dab his favorite fragrance between my breasts and behind my knees. I suppress an urge to dive into bed and stay until he relents, but he is struggling. I don't want to provoke upset, or add difficulty to his day.

When Randall breezes through in an evening suit, I race after him down the narrow, carpeted stairs to the stuffy garage, and we drive away in his upmarket sedan. At the street, we pass flowering trees that have dropped all their blooms, the breeze-ruffled arcs of Buckingham Fountain in Grant Park, and the expansive green lawns that set off the boxy skyline etched black against a deep blue sky.

I ask as casually as I can, "When can we visit that meditative synagogue?"

Randall is silent. He darts in and out of the Saturday night traffic as if ready to run over our future to reach our destination. After an abrupt lane change he says, "I'd rather spend time with you."

"Thanks. But we can go there together, can't we?"

"It's Saturday," he says irritably. "And we have to eat."

His temper is short, and the traffic dangerous. I change the subject. "I sold more cases than usual today. Pappas Restaurant ordered two!"

Randall changes lanes distractedly and smiles crookedly. "There's your market. Pappas-made wines for Pappas-owned restaurants."

Randall is soon submerged in the exacting task of hurrying through sluggish traffic. I watch the blank expanse of water and remember happy views of Port Phillip Bay until we are beyond the Loop and Randall is parking near a handsome brick mansion reflected in a large pond. He puts a hand on the small of my back and rushes me up the stone front steps into a brightly lit, forest green lobby. A severely dressed, sour-mouthed hostess takes Randall's name and tells us to wait. While Randall watches to be sure that she takes us in turn, I join a few couples in sitting on the velvety banquette at the center that is topped by a huge vase of gaudy tropical flowers and lit by a pendant lamp. Soon the hostess escorts us to a high-backed half-moon booth that faces a set of French doors framing a million-dollar view of the curvilinear Hancock building.

I know that this grand view and our conventionally luxurious booth, which is intimate in its privacy, clean with crisp white linens, and romantically lit by low candlelight, is everything that it should be. I know that I am not. "Ma'am? Ma'am! Can I have a double martini right away?"

Our hostess' face shows irritation, but she replies with punctilious politeness, "I'll speak to the waiter."

"Thanks."

Randall gives me a dubious look. "Since when do you like martinis?"

"I don't."

After we slide sideways into our seats, and before Randall decides how to take my remark, a dignified, elderly waiter with white, slicked-back hair and a precise moustache glides to the table. He deposits a martini in front of me, then pulls a menu from under one arm and opens it for me with a flourish and a bow. He does the same for Randall, and promptly disappears like an exiting actor.

I take a swig of my drink and think wistfully of the humble elegance of the table Maman kept, and the charming ease of Reggie's. I reflect on the relative poverty of the farm and try to be grateful. Then I look at the menu and blurt, "Look at the prices! I could have made crêpes, and you could have invited a few friends for dinner, and we could get on with creating a shared life."

"Don't mind the cost. It's our one-month anniversary."

"Oh!" I am nearly persuaded that I should accept that this is what he likes when I notice he is staring at the tabletop candle rather than the view, and is fondling his fork instead of me. He is absent. He may be lost.

I scramble for the Zen state of no expectations. "Penny?"

Randall shakes his head. He will not share his thoughts. I have just run into the invisible barrier between us, which now feels smooth and cold.

The waiter returns. His black suit and white shirt hang loosely on his bones, as if his practice of the art of the table prevents him from eating. His brows and long nose form a cross that symbolizes gravitas and Old World service. As he recites the specials, his accent is like an appetizer, and his passion for the fish of the day piques our interest. When I order, he smiles sly approval and darts toward the kitchen like an ambassador with a message for the Pope.

"Every one of my patients was distraught today."

I recognize with relief that Randall is inviting me to share in his inner work. "I'm sorry to hear that. It must take a lot out of you."

"We've had anti-abortionists protesting all week. Today they got aggressive, shouted abuse, threw things."

"I didn't realize you did abortions."

"We don't. But another doc in the building still offers them. And they go after all the patients because they can't tell which are which."

"Why don't the patients talk to the protesters, tell them their stories, let them know their problems and how they feel?"

"Every one of them has a long and painful story that's no one else's business."

The cold, smooth barrier between us has dissolved just enough for us to touch each other, but it still blocks intimacy. After a pause, I ask, "Do you want to tell me yours?"

Randall starts, and then says disingenuously, sneaking a side-glance at my face. "I don't want to get too serious. It's a relief to be with someone who doesn't want to talk about fertility."

He's twisting the truth again. I'm beginning to lose track of the real. I'm getting confused.

My breath catches. My equanimity falters. I clutch my napkin. I force myself to speak. "That's not quite true," I begin, trying to find the right words. "I want to talk about our vision, and our purpose."

"I have regrets!" Randall confesses abruptly. He moves as if to meet my gaze and then turns to stare absently at the skyline. "When I was in high school, well, she was young and I was young, and our parents wanted it over, and her family moved, and I never saw her again. But now I worry, you'll understand this, that the soul that chose us was—is—scarred, or homeless, or..."

I stare at the grid of lighted windows that form geometric patterns on the skyscrapers behind which the night sky is losing its last touch of heavenly blue. Faint strains of the Brandenburg Concerto drift into the space between our booth and the French windows. My mind begins to fill the crossword puzzle of lighted windows with explanations for his avoidance of our shared future, and of the unborn realm we touched in the Yarra. *A lost conception. A life dedicated to infertility. A painful marriage. A loss of sexual confidence. A custody battle. A loss of faith in the uncreated.*

Randall whispers, "I've never told anyone about that before."

"You've more than atoned through your work. It's time to forgive yourself."

"Do you forgive me?" He fixes my gaze with a wordless plea.

"There is nothing to forgive. Unless you punish us both by giving up on our shared future, and the new life that was coming into being through us, whatever form it might take."

Randall sucks in a breath and interrupts. "I've lost the girls."

"What?"

"The custody decision came down today. I have no rights."

He squeezes my hand so hard it hurts. My breath comes quickly. The cold hard barrier between us is gone. He barely confided in me all month, and now is letting loose all at once. I am barely keeping up. I down my martini. The burn of the booze wakes me to the fact that this is what I have been waiting for. We are doing the work now, the inner work that comes to us through him but belongs to both of us.

When the waiter has delivered a plate of garlic-dotted Brie and turned it to the precise angle that enhances its presentation, my linear thinking comes back online. "How? You had a great lawyer."

"She bought a better one. And—and—" He stops and tenses.

"Tell me. We need to share it. All of it."

"My junior partner's wife testified that I abandoned the girls for a vacation in Australia, and that I'd been experimenting with tantric sex, and that I brought you home to cohabit, and they made me out to be an irresponsible pervert. And then they said I'd risked the girls' lives by taking them in to work when the protesters were there. And then they put the last nails in the coffin by persuading the judge that I was reckless and stupid too."

"Those are lies, and we both know it. You do know it, don't you?"

Randall shakes his head. That cold smooth barrier rises again, sustained by the tension transmitted by his clenched hand. I see it now. He is punishing himself with blame, and punishing me, too. The beauty in our shared purpose has disappeared behind the curse visited on him by legalism and its ability to call on common prejudices when taking vengeance on a target. He is separating himself from the blessings of consort practice. He feels betrayed by his interest in sacred sexuality, and in me.

I say, "This isn't justice. This isn't what Solomon would do. We should be grieving for the harm this will do to you and your girls, not celebrating like this."

"Appearances are everything. If virtue doesn't show, well, it doesn't exist."

"That's only true in the tabloid version of reality."

"People will believe anything about gynecologists. All it takes is a vindictive ex, a lawyer who can rationalize anything, and a persuasive story."

"You need Rabbi Benji now. He can give you guidance that suits you, guide you through the valley of shadows, help you bridge your old life to our new one."

He makes no reply. I hold his hand, and I invite the invisible hearse of his first fatherhood to pass us, followed by the curses that walk behind like mourners collecting blood money. I wait and listen with my body for an opening in the wall he has constructed, but feel only a new wave of tension, and the dry sob that shakes his ribs. With his next breath he confesses, "I tried to offset the early error with my work. And I came to terms with my temper. But it was too late. And now I have to pay the piper."

I wait. I try to be patient while Randall pores over his napkin as if considering alternate vowels for unwritten syllables. When the waiter passes by to remove our barely-touched appetizer plates, Randall adds in a raw voice, "I worry that that soul, or another soul, might choose me before I'm ready."

The wall falls. I can see, now, that he has taken on too much, that he wants me but is not ready for me. I want to tell him that I will help with every trouble he has opened up, and any that remain hidden or have yet to come. I want to tell him that there is no hurry, that he should take whatever time he needs. But I can't say those things in honesty. I am giving way under the weight of his baggage. Soon I will be emptied of purpose, and of no use to anyone. I tell myself to give this experiment one more month. If we have not envisioned a purposeful life, and taken a first step toward it, I will go.

Randall adds, "I can't afford to buckle now. It was nothing I didn't expect."

"I'll never forget that you opened up to me like this tonight."

Randall looks at me warily. He laughs a single, sarcastic ejaculation, and then teases me. "My, we're portentous tonight!"

"The good news is we're facing the tough stuff, which is what we intended to do together. It's what our practice is for."

The waiter arrives with our main courses. Randall releases my hand, and we turn our attention to the meal. We admire its presentation, discuss its textures, and speculate on which wine might best enhance each flavor. We listen to the music in the background and try to identify it, and remember our favorite books and walks. Randall points to buildings in the skyline and tells me their history as if he feels pride of ownership in their architecture. When the dessert arrives, and we have nearly recovered our spirits, he says, "This is tantra, too, at least in the Hindu tradition, which nurtures pleasure in all the arts of life."

"I'm glad you said that. I thought we might have lost track of the sacred."

Randall frowns and changes the subject. "I have another surprise—"

But before he can finish, a tall woman who appears to be the perfect trophy wife appears at our booth. Randall stands so hurriedly that his napkin slips to the floor. He shakes her hand.

"I just wanted to say hello and thank you," she says in a throaty voice. She holds his hand in both of hers until my heart is pounding like a war drum and I feel an irrational and unwanted loathing of her silky blond hair, sun-browned skin, and the mauve silk dress that glides over the trim lines of her sculpted figure, revealing its allure without showing its flaws.

A man appears at her side and puts his arm protectively on her shoulder. His graying temples and hand-tailored Italian suit accentuate his aura of power and privilege. "Dr. Noll, a pleasure. What would we have done without you?"

When they leave, Randall sits down, stabs a piece of chocolate decadence with his fork, and dabs it daintily in his cream.

"Who was that?"

"A patient. I rarely go out without running into one."

"She was pretty chummy."

"When you treat infertility, you become a part of someone's life."

"If you had introduced me, what would you have said?"

"I wouldn't. It's professional, not personal. I'm the best in my field, not a public figure with a public consort." Randall finishes his cake, dabs his mouth with his still-crisp napkin, and grins wickedly.

"You like making me jealous!"

"Earlier you said you'd always remember me. Like you had one foot out the door. I could use the reassurance."

"Do you really want me to stay?" I blurt in surprise.

Randall's face opens in mirrored surprise. He grasps my hand again, this time so tightly it hurts. "How can you doubt it?"

"You never ask me what I want. You never sleep in my chamber."

Randall's lower lip presses upward in an expression I've never seen. He is so angry he can't divert his feelings into his pool of ever-present tension.

I add, "I want to be supportive, and grateful, and to share your burdens. But I care about my life too."

"You have all the time in the world."

"But I don't have you, or a community."

"What about your job, and your yoga class, and the condo?"

"You're providing every material good I could wish for, and I'm grateful, but I'm as isolated as I've ever been."

"Why? Who's stopping you from making friends?"

A blot of shame spreads through my chest. If we escalate unhappiness like this, in a cycle of blame and shame, we are bound to fail. I try to rally, and to cut off the cycle.

"I'm not blaming anyone. I'm only pointing out that I can't keep going as we are, with no shared vision. I simply don't have the strength, and if I did, I wouldn't want to use it to perpetuate a life that makes you unhappy."

"It's all I can do to keep my head above water."

"You're choosing our work for both of us, and against my will."

"I can't just quit being a doctor. It's what I am. And we have bills. You can't pay them by selling wine to five restaurants."

"I'm sure you don't mean to buy my life with money."

Randall sighs in exasperation. "What do you want from me?"

"Respect and consideration. Not as a gift, or a luxury, but because you value me, and you can't wait to get home and get on with building our shared life."

Randall looks at his watch. He takes a deep breath and puts on a happy face. "We can talk about all of that later. We have another event to attend."

He stands abruptly. He's game ready already, and although tense enough to be as hard as a statue, he has the grace to arrange his jacket with a flourish and to smile with winning charm. I realize that I am smiling reflexively, as if he has persuaded me that if things look perfect, they'll feel that way. He puts up a palm in a silent signal that I should wait, and then disappears from view. I wait and wonder at how happy I am on the outside and how numb within. When Randall reappears a few minutes later, he says with astonishing energy, "I've got too much on my plate. But tonight, we're out on the town, and it's time for the next surprise."

I try to match his sanguine spirit. "The show must go on?"

"Absolutely," he declares with a knowing smile.

He wins me over completely. When we emerge from the door, a cab is idling at the bottom of the stairs. We get in, and the jumpy driver zooms away as if courting suicide. The cab speeds to the

Loop and jolts to a stop next to a brick building beneath a sign reading "Backroom." Randall pays with a generous tip, hands me out of the car, and extends his elbow with playful chivalry. I remember the man I fell in love with. I smile again, this time from the heart, and take his arm. We walk down a canvas-covered boardwalk, around a corner, and through a door that looks like a service entrance. It may date back to Prohibition, when gin joints flourished, and secrecy and bribery dominated the playbook for selling vice.

Inside, a skinny bouncer with scraggly hair and a large Adam's apple points his thumb to the dark main level, where we grope our way to an open café table beside the low stage. The rounded platform is like a music store overstocked with drums, keyboards, and horns. When the waitress has taken our drink orders, and the club is nearly full, the house lights go down; only four blue spotlights are left, illuminating four microphones.

An invisible emcee announces with pregnant pauses, "And now. Put your hands together. For Chicago's. Own. Bluebird!"

The audience claps enthusiastically. A quartet files on stage.

Randall whispers, "That's John with the sax."

John is tall, balding, and plain. Unlike Randall, he appears nondescript. That changes when he begins to play a variation of Miles Davis' "Blue." Then, his fingers caress the keys, his lips work the reed, and he coaxes out of the hard brass horn lyrical cascades of sensual, sexual phrases. The audience is transfixed. Randall puts his arm over my shoulder. I put my hand on his leg. We forget our cares. John plays with the ease of close conversation, the intensity and urgency of desire, and climaxes with the ecstasy of coupling. By the time he stops, we are drunk with desire that carries us all the way through the first set.

When it ends, John approaches. "Hey, glad you could make it."

Randall stands up, shakes his hand, and says, "This is Colette. She came back with me from Australia. She grew up with Melissa."

For a moment, John is paralyzed, and then he drops anchor into the empty chair across from me. He grasps my water glass and frowns at the slippery cubes. His knuckles whiten.

I turn to Randall and say pointedly, "Would you like to get some air?"

Randall's face assumes the everything's-under-control expression that he uses to conceal shock. He stands, gestures awkwardly toward the door, and wends his way through the desultory crowd.

"I talked to her today," I say, and then put my palm on the tufts of curly black hair that is sprouting from the back of John's right hand. "She said to tell you that she thinks of you always."

His throat makes a grating noise of disgust. "That's it?"

"If you'd heard her voice…you'd know how much she cares for you."

His shoulders tense visibly. After a pause he eases them slightly and says, "Didn't mean to be rude. Randall didn't say. I wasn't prepared."

"I'm sure she would have liked to say more, but she hasn't told me anything about you for decades, and I don't think she can, yet."

John stares at his hands for a moment and then stands to leave. I jump up and grab his arm, desperate to convey my friend's feelings. "Think of what you two have! With Randall, I know it won't last, but I have the chance to love him. And that means everything. Now and forever."

John's mouth disappears into a thin line. His eyes turn red. Suddenly he throws his arms around me, and I give prudence a holiday and press my body to his. I want to remind him of what it feels like to hold a woman in love. I realize too late that I have opened my body to the pain of a man with a broken heart. We stand for a time, bookends of romantic love, I representing its first blush and he its final loss. And then his body shifts subtly, and I feel something more urgent in both of us. I feel confused. I stand stock still until a chair scrapes behind me, and I turn to see Randall sitting at the table, eyeing us suspiciously.

John casts an aggressive glance at Randall and says edgily to me, "If you get tired of him, give me a call. That seems to be the routine."

Randall's shoulders slump. He says contritely, "Blue was great. What's next?"

"Hot jazz, Bossa Nova, Reggae, and Zydeco. The drummer sits in because we let him play what he wants, and he wants to play a little of everything!"

"What Zydeco are you playing?" I ask.

"BeauSoleil. *Zydeco Gris Gris.*"

"My brother and I did that last year! We don't speak Créole, so I had to get some of the lyrics by heart."

"Do you want to sing? We've been talking about adding a vocalist."

"Private concerts only," Randall interjects possessively.

"That would be great!" I reply with feeling.

John's reckless invitation is probably some kind of dig at Randall, but I am thrilled to have been invited to join in this impromptu fête, and am filled with new hope that my soul has arrived in this place at last. I trail John to the stage to meet the barefoot drummer Chad, who up close is even more mute and otherworldly than he appears from the audience, and who assents to my participation with a curt nod. He gives me a sample of rhythm, and then the plump, curly-haired keyboardist scowls and transposes a vocal harmony line to suit his adaptation of the accordion part. John asks me to drop the English verses in the middle and promises to invite me to the stage when the time comes, and to cue me in.

When I return to my seat, and try to take Randall's hand hopefully, he crosses his arms and frowns through the hot jazz. He soon forgets his grudge, though, and taps his fingers to the sweet bounce of Bossa Nova. He taps his toes to the Reggae and, by the time I join John on the stage, Randall is smiling at me with an expression torn between amusement and anxiety on my behalf.

I ignore him. I take the mic and study the crowd as the band plays the lead-in. I note and ignore the Goth couple kissing wildly in the back, and the lone drunk who put his hand down his trousers the minute I walked on. I come in on John's cue. At first I am nostalgic for dancing Acadians, but then I take delight in seeing shy Midwesterners sway to the rhythm. By the time I finish the first verse, I am in stage love with the Bluebird fans, who are more attentive than the usual fête crowds of picnicking families with screaming children and shouting adults.

During the instrumental, Chad adds two bars to his solo, which confuses the combo. I bring them back in by dropping an additional verse while they find their way. When I end with, "*Tout que'qu'un Créole crie pour Zydeco,*" John shoots me a grin, as does Chad. His bare teeth stick out like tumbled-down tombstones above tufted whiskers that remind me of unmown grass. Randall applauds with his hands over his head. When I return to my seat, he gives me a peck on the cheek. I am in musical heaven, and he has joined me in it.

When the second set ends, Randall and I bid John and his

fellow musicians goodbye with handshakes all around. A second taxi takes us north, this one meandering until Randall takes over and directs the driver like a New Yorker. When the cab is en route, I snuggle up to him on the hard seat and put my hand on his thigh. Reckless with wine and desire, I say, "If I followed the left-hand path, I could make love to John for Melissa. I'd do it now."

I expect Randall to be titillated, but when the cab has gone, and we have taken our seats in his car, he shifts into reverse and wheels out of the parking space so fast that the car skids. He accelerates to the exit, turns recklessly into fast traffic, and speeds northeast toward the Lake. As he wheels round a corner, he asks accusingly, "Were you serious about John?"

"I was just trying to get into the spirit of bar hopping. It's all about flirting with transgression, isn't it? Centerfolds, and sex being naughty, and all that?"

Randall says nothing.

"Isn't that what you wanted?"

"Not from you!"

My mind turns over like a jar of marbles. I try to figure out which ones to chase. "Are you seeing someone else? Is that why you're always late?"

"No! I'm done with all that."

I retort like a small child. "Yeah? Well I never started."

I feel a strong impulse to jump out of the car and run to Yarra Spur, where my choices were few, but my life was rich in purpose and meaning, and sexual tension never got the best of me. "I have to say, it felt good to hold someone who wanted to be held."

Randall squeals to a stop at a red light. "What's that supposed to mean?"

"Every morning I offer myself to you and every evening you reject me! I was more than ready to make love when you got home, but you didn't come into my room. You never do."

"You don't make offers, you make demands!"

I crack. I jump out of the door and bolt up the sidewalk in the direction of the stoplight, waving my hand for a cab. When I realize that I have very little cash, I swivel and run back the other way. The driver in the car behind Randall looks at me and locks her doors. I am fully aware of my absurdity and yet am too wrapped up in it to devise an alternative.

In the distance I spot a red light flashing above an intersection. There is a bar on every corner. Above them is a billboard mirage in which I picture Ronnie and Liz sitting in a glitzy and appealing bar. In this fantasy, they are having an adventure rather than a misadventure. I enter into it in my mind's eye. I sit at the bar and order a drink and find a man sitting next to me who is ready to take me out back and relieve my desire, after which I will be able to collect my wits and go back to Melbourne and the safety and simplicity of celibacy.

The only thing that seems wrong to me at this moment, as I am running with unexpected agility in my red sandals, is that I am wearing the opal earrings that Randall bought for me. I should return them before I go.

"Colette! Colette! Where are you—Stop! Stop!"

I hear footfalls overtaking me. The mirage disappears, leaving a run-down street corner with seedy bars. I stop in confusion.

"Don't run away from me!"

I wonder how I got to this ridiculous point. I fold my arms in resolute befuddlement.

"Don't you like to go out on Saturdays?" Randall asks in surprise.

I start to laugh. I can't stop. I laugh, and laugh, and laugh and wonder at why we try to communicate, and how we could ever have had the crazy notion that we might think as one. When my crazy laugh subsides, I say, "I need to make love to a warm body right now. Any body would do. I've made myself ready for you over and over until I'm like a sexual volcano waiting to blow."

Randall puts his arms around me. He is laughing too, now. "Give me another chance? You'll like the next surprise. I know you will."

"You're sure it's for me and not for you?"

"It's for both of us. Equally."

"Just keep in mind that I feel rejected and thwarted sexually and emotionally, and that I can't take any more of it without losing my marbles."

He takes my arm gently and leads me to the car, which is sitting at a bus stop with its lights flashing like a squad car with an escaped suspect. I get in and sit in numb resignation. As he drives away, I see that Randall is oddly excited, as if our chase was an aphrodisiac. After a few long, silent blocks, he turns into the huge lot at Belmont Marina and parks the car in a vacant space.

"And now, the last surprise!" he says enthusiastically, as if he believes that this next scheme is going to make us forget the troubles he told me, or our inability to move on together, or the chance that this visit will end in scalding disappointment, heartbreak, and years of slow and painful recovery.

When I step out of the sedan, he takes off his tie and puts it over my eyes like a blindfold. In this deeper darkness, I notice the sounds of waves lapping gently and sails ruffling in the wind. He spins me three times, puts an arm tightly around my shoulder, and leads me toward the sloshing sound of boats at anchor. I forget my frustration in the confusion of orienting my body by sound and feel. Our footsteps sound like steel drums. Around us, lines creak and voices reverberate. I form an image of boat hulls and rocking sails. We are walking on a dock. When we turn, the air turns into a sea of disorienting echoes punctuated by raucous laughter. I lean dizzily into Randall and lose track of our direction. I feel his body and our desire and wonder whether he is about to plunge us both into deep water.

Suddenly he stops and pulls off the blindfold. We are standing on a lighted dock facing the stern of a cabin cruiser. Its sleek white surfaces reflect the city's glow. Beyond the covered stern deck sits a spacious cabin and a set of stairs leading to the bow. Around us, hundreds of boats pull dumbly at their lines.

"My partner's motor cruiser. Don't mind the drunks in the other boats." Randall jumps over the rail and hands me in.

"You sure you know how to pilot this?" I ask, holding a chrome rail to steady myself against the boat's yawing.

"Never had a problem before." He dances across the deck to open the cabin doors, sets a folding chair in the center of the stern deck, and motions for me to sit in it.

"What are we doing? This isn't grieving, or transformation. It's pretending."

"Just relax while I ready the boat. Two minutes."

I sit and stare at the dock, my mind a near blank. Randall jumps onto the dock, frees the lines, and jumps in again. He kicks off his dress shoes and socks, and after handing himself along the wood trim of the canopy like a monkey, swings himself up the narrow stairs. I hear the motor sputter, smell gas fumes, and feel the boat pull slowly away from the dock. Randall is steering us toward a vast wall of darkness. Five minutes later we pass a breakwater, and speed up until the boat is pitching across a washboard of waves.

When we have gone out several hundred yards, he shouts, "How do you like the view?"

The buildings of the Loop and north side are just beginning to merge into a single skyline profile. "I like it," I shout back.

"Come on up!"

I stagger past the cabin and up the stairs, where I plop down by Randall's side on a thick blue pad. We are on a bench behind the wheel. Randall veers and steers until the ride becomes slow and smooth. Then he sits back, puts his arm around me, drapes a soft plaid wool blanket over our shoulders, and looks up at the tiny glowing holes in the velvety night. Green and red pinpricks on the horizon mark distant boats. We are rolling gently on low swells raised by a light breeze.

Randall pulls me gently across his lap. My knees press into the cold foam bench pad. He pulls off my dress and chemise and puts the blanket around my back so that we are cocooned between the boat and the freshening air. I open his fly and take him inside. I move slowly, in near sync with the vessel's motion. Desire rises quickly. We make no effort to slow our release. I fall onto the seat beside him and pull the blanket around us.

I want to be his consort and his life partner. I think he wants that, too.

You're deluding yourself. It's slipping away like the shore.

He wants me, and he wants to have a baby with me to replace his children. I know he does.

So conceive his baby and leave him behind. Force him to choose between his old life and a new one with you. He'll have to choose you, or nothing.

I can't do that to him, or to a child. And he has plenty of choices, and hasn't chosen me.

Then why not be satisfied to have had a glorious affair, and move on?

I'm not ready. He was keen when I arrived; he may become keen again.

If you're his consort, you'll know what to do. If you can't figure it out, it wasn't meant to be.

I say, "This fast sex is like taking our hands off the steering wheel and letting inertia set our course."

"Profane love is the kind I know best."

"Change is difficult. But you don't really have a choice."

"I'm pessimistic now. About everything," Randall says. His face is hidden in darkness but his voice reveals regret.

"Don't give in," I whisper, kissing his soft neck. "If we aren't happy, we'll have no one to blame but us."

"Promise me you won't let anyone waste you. Not even me. Promise!"

"I promise. I'll stay strong. For both of us."

We sit side-by-side, hand-in-hand, and drift in no particular direction between the water and the stars, confusion and clarity, desire and purpose.

8

Strength

"Do you remember when I told you that the position might be temporary?" asks the saucer-eyed Mr. Garrity.

We are standing in his Printer's Row wine shop, which is laid out like a railroad car bisected by a double-sided display rack. Unlike the rotten fruit and dry hay smell of the tasting room at Yarra Spur, which reminded me of the bush land around us, this tasting room is industrial. It's dominated by the pulsating air conditioner and the greased metal shelves, which remind me of the printer's shops that used to thrive in this place. His shop gives off the cold, hard feel of a bottle morgue.

"Yes," says Mr. Garrity with a forced smile. "I'm going to have to cut back. I found a young man to work the noon hour."

The uncertainty of wine sales has turned this shy and fastidious man into a spigot of anxiety pressured by an inexhaustible hell of regret. He copes by tippling in the back room, and by inviting beautiful young men to work for him in the shop while he is there. This strategy has propelled the business into a slow downward spiral that he ascribes to a dip in the market. Randall's schedule being what it is, I offered to work from noon into the early evening, when the street is busy, but Mr. Garrity seemed to think that I was overstepping the bounds of a retail clerk.

"Business isn't what it was," he says. Taking a folded handkerchief from his back pocket to dab his moist forehead, he adds disingenuously, "I'm sure it's not your fault. And I'm sure your friend will take care of you."

When Mr. Garrity has written me a final check, I escape into the brick canyon of Dearborn Street and cross to the paved park on its sunny side, where I idle by cement-potted trees like a street-corner kid. I gaze at steaming puddles that add to the tropical July humidity, and watch waves of homeward-bound workers pass by. I wish them well in unloading the day's stockpile of stress and wonder what they might do for money.

I try to accept my rejection with equanimity. Randall has taught me well; I am glad to be gone the self-defeatist atmosphere of Mr. Garrity's shop, but I enjoyed meeting his customers and I will miss them. I will be one step farther from community and one step closer to the pall of lonely anomie. I try to put on the mind of Carl Sandburg, who saw this city's stockyards as hogbutcher to the world, and loved it just as it was. I try to be like Richard Wright, who encountered the worst of willful, hateful ignorance in this fractured society, and yet opened his big heart to do what he could to mend the abused and broken spirits that linger in this inner city.

I turn away from the ambitious young bloods hurrying past the park, hike my sport bag up my shoulder, and dart in the direction of a sandwich board with a big OM at the top. As I reach the ancient green-painted door and ascend the creaking staircase of the Sun and Moon Yoga Center, my body recalls that in the first week after my arrival, when I felt cold stress contract me and blind efficiency pull me, I took refuge in this center, where time is not everything and life is more than a race to the end of the day. I breathe deeply and let my body return to the state it had learned in the Yarra, and refresh my ability to delight in the grand panorama of unfolding time.

At the top of the stairs I join the long line of students waiting in a narrow, high-ceilinged hall to pay Grace, our trim, gray-haired teacher. She presides over her green metal cash box like a gatekeeper with a radiant smile. I enjoy the brief, personal check-in before we all turn inward and hide behind a wall of Midwestern reserve.

When I have changed my clothes in the small ladies' room and retrieved a block and mat from a side storeroom, I choose an open space at the front of the hushed studio and meditate on what V.S. Naipaul calls the great mixing of peoples, which brought yoga from India to this time and place. As I am meditating, a thought bubbles up from my gut. I recognize with surprise that I feel greatly relieved to not have to return to Mr. Garrity's shop, and when I open to the reasons for this unexpected joy at what I had taken as a rejection, I realize to my dismay that my work was only enabling the drinking, dissatisfaction, and decline of my employer.

Before I am able to integrate this revelation into my under-standing, Grace comes in and takes her place at the front of the room. We bring our palms together in front of our hearts to bow and say "*Namaste*," which Grace translates as, "the divine in me recognizes the divine in you." She fills the air with sweet words of peace that enfold us in kindness and open the door to beauty. It is easier, now, to hold the extremes of harm and hope in my heart, and to relax into turning the negative into the positive. I notice that the ceiling fans that revolve above us derive from trees and rock strata and also from the kind workers who made these wooden blades and metal fixtures. For the next hour, we attune our bodies to the sacred and beloved. At the end of class, we lie refreshed on our mats with our eyes closed. I see Randall's joy-filled face at Hal's seder, the Knife Edge of Mount Katahdin on my first Fourth of July in Maine, the ham-and-gruyere crepes with which Maman pleased Da, and myself sitting in meditation with Reggie.

When it is over, and time to return our borrowed goods, I realize that if I were back at Yarra Spur with Reggie I could feel this joy-filled abundance every day rather than for one hour three times a week. I resolve to try again to find a community here with which to grow in spirit. I join the neat line of students waiting to speak to Grace after class, and when my turn comes, ask, "Where can I learn to practice tantra?"

Grace smiles beatifically. "That is what we do here, in this class. We learn to transform ourselves."

"I mean, how can I take it off the mat and into my life as karma yoga? How can I find a community of people who do the work every day, around the clock?"

"We have a retreat coming up in a lovely place near Cancun."

I see that every door I open leads to an opportunity to buy a service rather than a chance to join a community of like-minded seekers. I know that she needs to make a living, but I am not looking for a cash transaction. "I don't want to buy it, or to do it now and then, I want to be it, and live it. I want to be a tantrika."

"In the last few sessions I'll talk more about taking our practice off the mat, and in the fall we may offer a weekly meditation class."

"I was hoping to find community here and now, somewhere in the city."

"Do you want to become a teacher?" she asks dubiously.

Apparently my asanas are not the best. I am not surprised. As much as I enjoy the body-grounded discipline of yoga, and the chance to drop in on an ethereal group-mind, I've never seen myself in Gracie's seat.

156

"What I really came to Chicago to do was to practice tantric sex like my friends in Australia."

Grace's beautiful smile disappears. She looks ten years older. "Many people have misconceptions about the purpose of tantra."

"Too true. All the more reason to find a qualified teacher."

"Why don't you try the Dharma Center?"

My heart sinks. I have tried many places, including the Dharma Center, where a cool, orange-robed monk spoke aversively about degenerate times. I tried a Siddha Yoga Center, where I chanted the *Guru Gita* with blind devotion. I tried a Gurdjieff group dominated by an opinionated organizer; a class in sacred turning offered by dour Sufis; and a retreat center for former Catholics who lied to each other as they had learned to do in confession.

Wherever I go, I think of Reggie, and realize that our meeting was a rare and precious opportunity to bask in grace and challenge. I realize that I miss her friendship, the organic wholeness of her life, and the teachings that I gleaned from her examples in everyday life—such as the way she spoke directly to the heart, treated complex notions and conventions as transparent tools for happiness, and practiced continually. I found in her a beloved life teacher for whom there can be no substitute. Being away from her exacts a price.

I persist. "I've been to the Dharma Center, and to so many other places, and talked to many, many people, but either they don't know or won't say."

Grace looks distressed. Perhaps she doesn't know, or doesn't want to break a sacred vow of secrecy. Either way, I must accept her answers. "Thank you so much for your class," I say. "I'd be lost without it."

I carefully return my borrowed things to the shelves at the

back, and try to catch up with Delia, the one fellow student with whom I've managed to connect, and who usually has coffee with me after class at a nearby café. I spot her brown braids at the bottom of the stairs, and reach her just as she is saying goodbye to another student. I notice that she is speaking in a fake Australian accent, and that her manner changes abruptly when she sees me.

As we walk toward the café, sweating off the heat of our yoga workouts, I ask, "What was that all about?"

"What do you mean?" she asks.

"The fake Aussie accent, and the in-your-face personality you put on."

She looks at me as if sizing me up for a story, and then she seems to drop the personality that she usually puts on for me. "I'm an actress. I try different characters."

"Which one are you usually doing with me?"

"I try to mimic you. I do you."

"Why?"

"I'm an actress. I practice whenever I can."

I say nothing as we enter the café, line up for coffee, and take seats at the front window, side-by-side. I can't imagine why she would behave as a chameleon, mimicking people indiscriminately, playing with their inner and outer forms without respect or regard. I wonder if it is ethical. I wonder if it is sane. This time, as I sip my iced coffee, I watch her instead of the passersby.

"You might want to work on the Aussie accent," I say.

"Why?"

"It's not Aussie, or kiwi, or South African. An Aussie would know."

"How do you know?"

"I lived there for a while."

"Can you do it for me?"

"No, sorry. Don't have that talent, or skill. Whatever it is."

She looks irritated. I have the feeling that I am seeing her for the first time—that until now I have been talking with her characters, and not with her. I wonder how she might behave when she is doing herself.

"What are you doing here?" she demands.

"I think I mentioned that I came back to spend time with a man I met. And I've been working, too, but I lost my job today. Which is fine."

She looks at me like a carnie spotting a mark. "How will you get by?"

"My … friend … is paying for the class, and this coffee. I won't have to worry."

I have told her all of this before. I wonder if she has forgotten it, or if she is buying time, or perhaps forming a new character.

"In ancient times," Delia says, "people worshipped goddesses, and priestesses ran temples for ritual sex. And then Roman soldiers spread a culture of rape. And now in our commercial culture, sex is all about money. Which means that it's about prostitution."

I struggle with shame. I don't know what may have happened to her in the past, but I'm fairly sure that she is trying to wound or anger me. "That's terribly cynical."

She looks disappointed, perhaps because she cannot see or enjoy the hurt that she has caused. She continues confidentially, "Whenever I get a female role, and I play it like a virgin or a prostitute, I sell tickets. If I play a spiritual woman, or an ethical one, or a leader, no one wants to see it. Which is why I like to do you when I'm with you."

"Can you do kindness? Fake it, I mean."

"I don't fake anything!" she objects. "An emotion like that

is a state of being. You're it, or you're not."

"Can you be it?"

"I can use the method to become it."

"Can you show me?"

She tries on characters like some women try on dresses. She asks for my opinion, and takes it well when I point out flavors of false kindness, like unctuousness, approval seeking, smirking, sensuality, and condescension. It becomes a game. I begin to enjoy it, and to see the wisdom that she could glean from being the character and watching the reactions. In her falsity, she is closer to reality than anyone else I have met here. In this interplay, this dance of playful pretense, we are touching on the uncreated that I had hoped to explore with Randall. Delia and I end our encounter in laughter, and take our leave as soul friends who can practice in parallel, if not in unison or in dialogue.

I shoulder my bag and return reluctantly to the sweltering heat outside. I notice sunlight sparkling on an oil slick in the gutter, and follow its reflected rays to the bell of a saxophone played by a bearded musician in a battered pork pie hat. The case beside him is open in an invitation to commercial community. I stand at the edge of the sidewalk and watch. His eyes are closed. He is in a land I cannot see, and yet we form an island in a river of commuters. I wonder if I could be in it and yet apart from it as he is, and whether if I busked I might find my community, or form a continuous practice in everyday life. I cannot picture it. I see myself alone in a crowd.

Randall is the only reason I'm here, and he doesn't have time for me.

Face it. He's lost interest.

This is a hard time for him.

How hard could it be to come into my chamber and lie down?

He acts like I'm forcing him to spend time away from work.

Reggie was right. His heart's a stone.

If you could open it for him, or with him, it would have happened by now.

Ten brooding minutes later, when I cross the patch of dark green sod under the spindly tree in front of the condo, I spot an unfamiliar British-made sedan in the driveway. The front door opens, and Randall calls out to me in displeasure, "Where have you been?"

"At yoga class. The one I've been taking for six weeks?"

"I thought we agreed to be home by five on Fridays."

"You get home at six or seven, so I started going to the Friday class."

"These guys work so hard," says a nasal voice. "And they should. We need the money." A skeletally thin woman appears next to Randall. She seems to be in her late twenties, and is wearing thick red hair, a tiny dress, dark make-up, and heavy jewelry. "Rachel Steiner. Good to meet you. Finally. Randall wrapped you in mystery. Come in and meet my David."

I toss off my shoes and follow her into the sky-lit foyer, where the cold slate floor of the formal living room offers welcome cooling. I realize with a chill that she is the woman who testified against Randall in the custody battle. I put on my most formal politeness. "I'm sorry to have kept you waiting. I didn't know you would be coming."

"David is Randall's partner."

"Yes, I'm aware of that."

"We would have had you over, but David's been so busy. We should have you up to the lake for a ride on the new jet skis. We'll do it soon."

David, a tall man with deep brown eyes and a heavy unibrow,

stands up from his seat on the couch to squeeze my hand. His take-charge look and ease tell me that he and Rachel have spent more time in Randall's living room than I have. Their practiced smiles say that they are all trying to pretend the custody battle did not damage their friendships. "Pleased to meet you."

Randall says, "I invited David and Rachel to have drinks at Solaris. They can't make the concert."

"What concert is that?"

"The one at the park. With Stan and Ellie."

"I don't like to drink below the 34th floor," Rachel interjects. "And I never eat outside."

"Let Colette have her shower," David says in an aside to Randall. "Women need their primping."

I try to ignore his condescension. When I finish my shower, I hear a car start and drive away. I race into the living room. Randall is standing with his arms folded, looking out at the street.

"I tried to be quick. I never thought they'd leave!" I exclaimed.

"They're meeting us at Solaris."

"They're driving? It's only a few blocks. And it's impossible to park!"

Randall puts his hands up, signaling me to stop. "David and I get along by keeping our opinions to ourselves."

We walk quickly to Printer's Row, keeping to the shade where we can. Randall explains that he has planned a full evening, and that after having drinks with David and Rachel, we will have dinner in the park with his senior partner, Stan, and his wife Ellie, and then meet his old college friends Sarah and Doug in Hyde Park.

"I've been here three months. Why am I meeting everyone tonight?"

"Don't worry. Stan and Ellie are very religious and Doug and

Sarah are very sexual. They make your favorite combination."

"I'm just wondering why you didn't mention it."

"I figured you didn't have another date."

Randall gives me a winsome smile. As we approach Solaris, he puts a hand protectively behind my back. When we arrive at the door of a corner bar that is topped by a huge carving of a smiling sun, he ushers me gently inside. His hand communicates tension that fills me until my body forgets yoga class and the strange practice with the actress. I am back in a state that is like stress worship, and that my body would rather reject than transform.

"I should warn you. Rachel is very close to my ex-wife."

"Let's send her our love," I say ironically.

Randall tenses and eyes me suspiciously. We pass a greeting sign that says, "Seat Yourself." He scans the cavernous interior, which was once home to a pressroom, and then we take a high wooden table against the far wall. While we wait, we say little, and look at each other less. I feel a powerful surge of blame that may be coming from Randall, or from me. We both know that it is Rachel who enabled Randall's ex Jenny to take the girls, and who appears unaware of the damage she has done.

When Rachel and David have entered and spotted us, and while they are still ten feet away, Rachel begins to crow over David's no-cost parking space. When she sits down, she starts to grill me.

"So, are you two buying a house?"

"Randall already owns a home."

"You know what I mean, a family house."

"I'll have to get back to you on that."

"Do you have children? You're a little old to start a family."

Accepting that she will not be deterred, I gamble on a blunt reply. "It isn't up to me alone. Unlike some women, I think a child has a right to her father."

Rachel's face twists. She and David glance apprehensively at Randall, whose face has closed. Rachel holds up her palms to signal stop. I realize that this gesture, which Randall so often uses, may come to both Randall and Rachel through the ex-wife I have never seen. "I agree with you. Enough said."

I contain my astonishment and ask, "Do you have children?"

David says proudly, "Rachel has a career."

"We have to have a lot more money before I have a baby. The Latin School costs as much as college! And we have so many expenses! And we need a four-wheel drive car in case we want to go up to the lake house in winter, and we can only update the kitchen and bathroom if I get more clients. And I want to go to St. Lucia for the holidays."

"It seems like everything's getting so complicated," I say evenly.

"You're so right! And there are so many memes out there! It's getting harder and harder for me to get my clients' messages out. I specialize in markets for children under ten. They're the easiest. Television reaches all of them."

"Rachel's in marketing," David explains. "It's a good field for women."

"David! Most of my colleagues are gay men!"

"As I was saying," David replies.

"Can a gay man be the mother of your children?"

Rachel cranes her neck around the room and launches into a critique of its décor. Her least favorite wall hanging is the pub's T-shirt, a black cotton shirt featuring a shiny gold sun wreathed by Celtic knots. As she gapes at it, her face is a rising barometer of determination.

When the waitress arrives to take our drink orders, Rachel says, "I want to talk to the manager."

Within minutes, a burly red-haired man with a ponytail, beard, and elaborate tattoos comes from the back and strides toward our table. I think he is a bouncer until he says, "I'm the owner. What can I do for you?"

"You should be full by this time of day. I could do a survey for you to find out what people want for happy hour."

"I don't want to be full now. I want to be full at two. And I will be." A smirk simmers at the edges of his wide nostrils.

"You could increase your profit margin substantially if you offered the public what they want."

"I offer what I want and make a good living at it. Is that all?"

Rachel purrs seductively. "If you're making the profit you want, then you're doing exactly the right thing."

The waitress arrives with our drinks. The owner lets Rachel off with a smile of gruff charisma. "Enjoy your drinks. Come back if you like them."

After he leaves, Rachel says, "So few businessmen understand marketing!"

I sip my margarita and say, "He understands profit. This is all water."

"This is what I'm saying! He should know what you, the customer, would like in a bar."

"If he tried to appeal to everyone, the bar would have no character. People would lose interest." I see that I am talking about Randall and me. I look at him and add pointedly, "Like a relationship without a shared vision."

The affinities around the table shift. Rachel looks at David and says, "We're both Jewish, so we know who we are and what we want." She looks at Randall. "What about you?"

"Yes, Randall, what about you? And me?" I probe.

"We like to have great sex on your boat," Randall says to David.

Rachel shoots a glance at David, who discovers a sudden interest in the T-shirt fixed to the wall above the table.

"Don't worry," I say. "It's the kind of profane sex you think of as normal, not the sacred sex you consider perverted."

"You're not Jewish. How could it be sacred?"

"Good question. If you had asked before giving testimony, you might not have made such a big mistake."

Rachel rolls her eyes. "They asked me a question, and I answered them. What was I supposed to do? Lie?"

"Are you saying that you were just following orders?"

Both Rachel and David flinch at this reference to the self-justification preferred by the perpetrators of the Holocaust—now called the Shoah. I have their attention now. A moment has opened in which to break the ice beneath the surface. I continue, "When you realize that you were used as a tool, you can regret the past and apologize. If you do it soon, we can get on with our lives, maybe even allow the girls to know their amazing father."

They are not ready. Randall is so angry that his voice is barely in control, and his face shows a fleeting expression of contempt. "Rachel's here as a courtesy to David. Let's be courteous to David."

The moment of possibility passes, and we resume our program loops, the ones that have been running our minds and our lives. Rachel snatches the drinks menu from behind the napkin dispenser and glares at it. "This design is terrible. They should have hired my friend Cindy."

The conversation thaws and turns to Chicago's political scandals. We rake the muck around Hizzoner da Mare's office beginning with the relatively recent collapse of a public parking garage, which was due to graft that left a gaping hole in the city's budget; and work our way back to Mayor Daley's beginnings in a Bridgeport street gang. When we finish, we all appear to be such perfect friends that I can hardly believe that as soon as we part, Rachel will rush to her car, pick up her car phone, and call Randall's ex so that they can run me down.

"That could have been much worse," I say to Randall as we walk to his home through the hot evening. "She probably thought she did the right thing."

"David knows who butters his bread. And so does Rachel."

"I don't know how you work with him when you feel that way."

"I'm his senior partner. It's their job to get along with us, not the other way around. Don't give it a second thought."

Apparently unable to follow his own advice, Randall frowns at the sidewalk and continues in silence. I try to sustain compassion for Rachel, but it is too easy for me to dislike her way of gathering money and her superficial but smug avoidance of pork and shrimp. I know Reggie would see pure light in Rachel, but I cannot do that, especially not while I am absorbing Randall's rage.

He and I brood as we fill a woven-wood picnic basket with fine French cheese, bread, and meat, and walk on in near silence to Grant Park carrying the basket between us like a cradle. It is weighed down with the absence of his daughters, the fruitlessness of my marriage, and the barrenness that he is choosing for us. It is exhausting to carry it all. I tire before we reach the stage located at Eleventh Street and Michigan Avenue, where a mass of brass, bows, and elbows sticks out of a tiny band shell.

We walk ten yards onto the grass and put down the basket. Randall scans the roiling crowd while I take in its gumbo of sounds and smells. Above the background noise of the orchestra tuning and the crowd conversing, we hear several Asian kindreds exchanging tonal shouts under the proscenium's lip, where they are sharing feasts doled out of multicolored plastic containers. Behind us, a bus disgorges a mass of young African Americans in purple robes who form rows below the exclamation mark of their conductor's baton and proceed to warm up with arpeggios.

Randall shouts, "Stan! Over here!"

I see a middle-aged couple standing twenty yards east of the band shell. Stan Rubin smiles brightly and waves. He is short and slight, and his face is a clay relic with huge features worn smooth. Ellie, who is shorter, is wearing an ill-fitting auburn wig that threatens to obscure her tiny features, which are already disappearing into matronly plumpness.

We converge and shake hands like doubles tennis players after a friendly match. I see a warm light in Ellie's eyes, and feel her mothering envelop us all. My heart rises as we find our way through the carpet of blankets holding the energetic couples and weary families who greet each other with complaints about traffic and the weather. When we reach an open space, Randall and I unfold his car blanket and pull it taut on top of the thick, crabgrass-rich lawn, which is damp with afternoon rain. The Rubins spread out a sandwich of waterproof tarp, worn sheet, and fluffy wool blankets.

Stan and Ellie are so genuine that in the first conversational lull, I decide to risk mixing humor with forthrightness. "Randall says you're the senior partner and it's my job to get on with you. I'm open to suggestions!"

Stan smiles shyly and looks at Randall, who shrugs helplessly. "Take care of Randall. He's like a son to me, or a little brother."

"Do you have children?"

"Five," answers Ellie. "They've gone to my brother's for Shabbos."

"We don't go out Friday nights," Stan adds, "But the last time Randall dragged me here we saw Solti conduct *Die Meistersinger,* and I'll never forget it!"

Having said that, Stan is done with social niceties. He looks up at the sky as if searching for the stars that herald the beginning of Shabbat. Finding none, he dives into a distracted argument, shaking his wild gray forelock as he makes his points, nearly catapulting his yarmulke onto a neighboring blanket. Randall engages with him in an intense discussion of a new method for pulling reluctant sperm into the gene pool. Beside us, a young man in a wrinkled suit, presumably unhappy to hear this talk of needles and testicles, takes his blanket and his date and goes in search of a new spot on the lawn.

"We need to use a needle with a bigger bore!" Stan insists.

"The problem is the stabilizer!" Randall counters.

"Let's go for a walk," Ellie says to me. Her eyebrows are low, as if sagging into a frown, which I discover is an indicator of her low level of interest in shop talk.

She and I make a circuit of Buckingham fountain, the waters of which drop abruptly, as if someone turned off the spigot. Ellie's eyebrows go up to the fringe of her wig. "So what are your intentions with our Randall?"

I smile. She is direct. I like that. "I promised to tend to him and love him. But he's disappeared into his work, and I can't tell if he'll ever come back."

Ellie clasps her hands together. "Randall's been having trouble at work. He's always worked too much, but now he's working longer hours and doing less. Stan says he's lost his focus. Again."

"Randall said he would take me to meet Rabbi Benji, but he hasn't done it, and I'm worried that it's because I'm not Jewish. What do you think?"

Ellie gives a one-shouldered shrug. She swerves to avoid a confluent group of blankets holding a group of elderly card-playing women. "When are you planning to convert?

"I'm not. I grew up Catholic, and it cured me of that."

Ellie makes a face of distaste. My heart sinks. I start to blather. "I know the laws mean a lot to you, but Randall says there are other ways of observing Judaism, and that he and I could make a spiritual life together."

Ellie looks insulted. I begin to believe that the conversation is over, but I plead, "You must see that it works differently for Randall than for you?"

"Since you brought it up, how does it work for Randall?"

The symphony strikes up Beethoven's Fifth, which makes our conversation sound both comical and doomed. "I don't know. When we met, we were both exploring spiritual practices. But now he doesn't take the time."

"He may be confused. He used to be entirely secular, like Jenny. Has he talked to you about her, and about his daughters Kyla and Krissie?"

"Hardly. It upsets him."

Ellie sighs tensely. "Jen has plenty of money of her own, and she would have spent it all on revenge, without a thought for the girls."

"It may be hard for Randall to work with David after Rachel's testimony."

"It may be hard for him to live with you after what Rachel said at the trial."

"Which was what? I didn't meet her until after."

"David tells her everything, and he shouldn't; he doesn't always understand it, and she's worse. She doesn't know how to deal with it like I do."

"Sometimes I worry that he's sorry we met."

"Do you love him?"

I put my hand over my mouth. My eyes fill with tears. I nod.

"You should convert. It isn't too late. Then you could marry, and Randall could know who he is again, and he could start over, if you're not too old."

I want to tell her that I'm lost and desperate for community, and so isolated that I'm losing my grip, and that I already wasted twenty years on a lost man, and that I'm nearly spent. It's time I took care of myself. It's time to put my life first. I want to tell her that I'd do anything for Randall, even convert, but that would be a lie, and this is no time for lies. I say nothing.

Ellie watches her clasped hands to avoid looking at a young couple entwined on a blanket. Then she sighs deeply. "We love Randall, and he loves you, so we love you too. So I'll tell you this, Jenny said no to Randall all the time, and someone has to say yes to him, at the right time, about the right things."

"If he doesn't get off the fence soon, I'll have no choice but to leave."

"And force him to choose."

"And to do what's right for both of us, and for the work we should be doing in the world as it is now. The *tikkun olam* we took on in Australia."

As we examine the decision that Randall and I have been putting off, Ellie says, "We have traditions about soul mates. Do you know them?"

"Randall says that soul mates were connected before the vessels of creation shattered and dispersed as divine sparks. Soul mates recognize the sparks in each other, and redeem them by reuniting them."

As we near our blankets again, Ellie says, "Anyone can be

your soul mate, and you can have many soul mates. Randall understands this. If he saw a spark in you, he won't forget it, and neither will you."

"Thank you for saying that. Rachel made it clear that she saw me as *treyf.*"

Ellie raises her eyebrows as if I have said a swear word and continues, "You see the way he is with Stan."

A few yards in front of us, Randall is propped up on one elbow with his legs sprawled out. His toes move in time to the music. Stan is hunched over his crossed legs staring intensely at the universe of ideas between his palms. Each is completely absorbed in their shared task. They are in union.

"There they are, *chesed* and *gevurah*, generosity and strength!" Ellie plops onto a patch of blanket next to Stan. I sit opposite Randall and listen to the orchestra wander through the darkness of Beethoven's soul. Later, when the *Ode to Joy* begins and the orchestra emerges into the light, Ellie sweeps her arm up toward the skyline and asks, "So, how do you like our great city?"

I look at the man-made cliffs of the Loop, behind which the bright red sky of sunset has given way to a midnight blue lampshade pricked by lights. "I like it. I used to come here when I was a girl. But I miss Melbourne. And I belong in the country."

"Randall liked Melbourne so much he tried to bring it home," Stan observes.

Randall and I look at each other wistfully. He opens the basket and cuts slices of pear and raclette cheese, and then baguette and triple crème. I recall the first time we shared these flavors. It was the day after we first made love. Remembering my manners, I say to Ellie, "Would you like some?"

I look at her just in time to see a flash of disgust at my offer of what she views as unclean. "Sorry," I mumble. I realize that even if

I grew to love Ellie and Stan as family, I would never be welcome in their kitchen and in their lives. If they knew Randall's roots, they might not welcome him either. I look at Randall sprawled out on the blanket and wonder at his confidence. Every day, he braves the judgment of loved ones and follows the spirit of the law as he sees it even as his trusted mentor, Stan, might judge and deny him. I wonder if Randall has struggled with the divine and attained the freedom of transcendence, or if some part of him sees me as other and unclean. As a former Catholic I have seen that a straitjacket of rules can sometimes work to free rare souls. But it is not a struggle that I would undertake. I would rather be conscientious, like Melissa.

When the concert ends, and the crowd disperses in all directions, Randall and I tote our basket to the Rubins' car, which is parked a few blocks away. I say sadly to Ellie, "It was nice to have met you two. Good-bye."

Ellie looks at me keenly and waggles her finger. "Never act in haste."

I walk back to Randall's condo holding up one side of the basket and holding in my feelings. Randall thought that I was portentous two months ago, when he took me out, and now it is true. The obstacles have piled up, and though we have named many of them, we have not faced them.

When we are back in Randall's kitchen he asks me, "What's wrong?"

I realize that I am swallowing back tears. "Long evening."

"Stan and Ellie are serious, but Doug and Sarah will be fun."

"Let's not go. Let's make love, and talk, and get on with our shared lives. I don't want to live your old life with you, especially without my consent. I've been too much of a pushover. I haven't been strong. And now I can't go on like this, with no shared vision. I just can't do it."

"Do we have to do this now?"

"I love you with all my heart. But I can't live with you like this."

"Colette, we can talk about this tomorrow. Right now, Sarah and Doug are waiting for us at the Medici Café in Hyde Park. We can't just let them sit there and wait for us, and not show up."

I try to gather and give him my strength. "I don't want to let you down."

"Let's go, then." His voice is triumphant.

I feel bullied. I doubt that he is taking a shortcut to make it through the night. I think he believes that he can make his life easy by crushing my will. Half an hour later, when he turns off Lake Shore Drive into Hyde Park, I realize that I have been thinking up a knitting project, a new throw with a complicated shell pattern. It is the first time I have done that since fleeing my old life by leaving Maine. I am moving backward into obedient oblivion. I am dangerously close to losing my way.

Randall parks the car. We walk thirty yards to a café with a distressed interior of bare brick walls, wooden beams, and graffiti. We pass between rows of high, rough booths and stop at a table. Randall stretches his arms out to the side. He is facing a woman with long blond hair, a straight nose, and well-defined arms. Her companion has a ponytail, stubbly beard, and the soft hulk of a former athlete. Randall puts his arm around my shoulder and says, "This is Colette! Colette, Sarah and Doug."

"Hi, Colette," Sarah says as I slide into the booth across from her. "So I heard you grew up with Melissa in Peoria but met Randall in Melbourne? How weird is that?"

"Not very," Doug interjects, "I'll bet you two cents Melissa put them together."

"Two cents? Not too confident," says Randall.

"Sarah can't bet in my league," says Doug.

"Sarah wouldn't bet against your wife's money," says Sarah.

"You mean against yourself?" I ask with a laugh.

"Oh, no," Sarah says with a wave of her hand. "We're not married. I mean—I'm not married to anyone, and Doug's married to someone else."

"Oh. I'm sorry. Randall said you'd been together for twenty years."

"Yup," Doug says. "We've been doing the dirty for twenty."

"On and off," Sarah adds. "He lives in California, and I live in New York."

"Are you happy with that arrangement?" I ask Sarah.

"I used to feel guilty, but you plan your life the best you can, and make mistakes, and things change, and you deal with it."

"Life is like long division. You get remainders. Like lovers who won't go away," Doug says with a wicked grin.

Doug elbows Sarah, and Sarah elbows him back.

He says theatrically, "Do it again, I love it when you hurt me."

"How much have you had to drink?" Randall asks Doug.

"Drink? Who drinks anymore?" Doug laughs. When no one else laughs, he sulks. "Okay, okay. Comedy is all in the timing."

Sarah explains soothingly, "Doug doesn't get to cut loose very often. When he's working through a big deal, he has to plan every little move; when he's with me he feels safe enough to say whatever he wants."

When the waitress has arrived, we order coffee and dessert, and Doug asks me, "So how is Miss M these days?"

"Melissa? She's doing well. I spoke to her this morning."

I tell a few stories of Melissa, and describe our night with

John's Bluebird group, which Sarah and Doug know and like. When our orders arrive, Randall and his friends share stories of campus life, and ask about our time in Australia and Chicago. They drift into serious topics, and offer sympathy and support on hearing Randall's news of his loss of visiting rights. And then, just as it seems that we are all getting on, Sarah and Doug lose interest in the conversation and go back to a cycle of escalating aggression smoothed now and again with loving words.

I am not surprised when they talk explicitly of the ways in which they arouse each other with aggression and pain, and of how difficult it is to know when they should end an episode of this potentially dangerous affair to keep it from getting out of hand. I notice that Randall is unperturbed by this news. I know that he has probably heard far worse in the course of his work, but these are friends, not patients, and I am distressed to know that he is at peace with their destructive pattern, and sometimes coldly amused by it. He is revealing patterns in himself that I would rather not see.

I remind myself not to judge. And then I remind myself that I do not want to use my energy for destruction, or for blocking out the pointless but deliberate pain of others. Rather than block out their energy, I try to take it in, and to direct it toward the destruction of my own bad patterns. I recognize to my dismay that it is obedience that I must purify.

Finally, I interrupt them to ask, "Doug, why do you stay in a job that makes your life so unpleasant?"

Doug looks at Randall incredulously. "I make a lot of loot, sister. *Beaucoup.*"

"And Sarah, why do you stay in a relationship that doesn't bring you joy?"

Sarah stops and frowns. She squints as if looking into the

distance. "Doug and I have chemistry that I can't forget. He has too little with his wife, and too much with me."

"And what about his wife?"

Sarah looks at Doug apprehensively.

Doug replies carelessly, "My body disgusts her, and I can do without hers."

"Why do you stay with her?"

"Where's the interrogation light?" Doug asks theatrically.

"She's only curious," Sarah says gently.

"My wife's my best friend and investment partner, and all our marriage needs is for Sarah to have sex with me. And now we're fine. We're all fine."

Sarah smiles genuinely and says, "You remind me of Melissa."

I return a rueful smile. "You mean judgmental?"

"No. And yes. She was our anchor back in the day, she and John together. When the four of us were together, we were all fine, really fine."

"Because we were talking about Randall's exploits," Doug interjects edgily.

Sarah stands and pulls Doug's sleeve. He rises grumbling, slams a twenty on the table, sneaks a scratchy kiss on my cheek, and walks toward the front door. Sarah lingers to take my hand and say, "I know this is a rough time, but you and Randall would be great together. I hope your visit turns out to be more than a rebound affair, and that you'll come and visit me. I'm studying to be a yoga instructor. We'd have a lot to talk about."

When they are both gone, Randall looks at me expectantly. I say, "That was a gracious invitation. I like her."

"She and Doug are hilarious together. And no matter what happens, they always find a way back to each other."

Randall tops up the small pile of cash on the table, and we

exit toward the door. As we walk to his car, I glance at his profile, and see by the streetlights that he seems content. When we drive away, I have the strange sense that he has merged with his purring sedan as completely as if he had engineered himself to enhance its lines and its function.

I turn away and gaze meditatively at the vast expanse of the Great Lake that is passing on our right. We seem to be in a road movie tracing the surface of a dark, wild planet. I remember that under the seeming blank of air and water, the depths are transforming human waste, redeeming it by turning it back into the raw materials of life. I hope that it isn't too late for us to do the same.

Gradually, my body discerns a pattern. It is not like an image or a phrase; it is a hologram of Randall's heart that my heart is recreating, one enclosed by a force field. He protects his heart from sorrows and schemes by creating a barrier that enables him to deal intimately and lovingly with pain and suffering. It is this very barrier that is barring him from the free exchange of mutual love. It is the source of all of the barriers that arise between us, and is fed by uncertainties about religion and vocation and by worries about identity and union.

"Did you notice that Doug and Sarah bring out the worst in each other?"

"You haven't known them very long. She's good for him."

"They make each other miserable. Each is the other's hell."

"I agree that their adultery is troubling. But it works for them."

"Did you notice that your problems, and theirs, and Melissa's are all similar, and that they haven't changed much in twenty years?"

"Everyone has problems."

"You wouldn't have said that when we were in Australia. You were ready then to embrace change, and to explore a new kind of life with me."

"You heard what Sarah said. This is rebound time. But we can weather it."

"We can't choose our past or our obstacles, but we can choose our response. You respond differently to things here than you did when I met you."

"We both knew it would be hard on us when I went back to work, but I'm holding steady now. I won't buckle."

I am at a loss for words. If inflexibility is holding him together, I do not want to undermine it. I do not want to break him. I put my mind to the problem. Randall is emotionally dissociated; he cannot detect the seeds of suffering, or distinguish sources of pain from sources of love and joy. He can barely read his own feelings, and is oblivious or hostile to mine. In Australia, away from his old life, he could. But now he is working blind.

"Maybe you should buckle. You're surrounded by people who you think don't know who you are. Maybe you're the one who doesn't know. And maybe you can't find out without letting the old façade fall. There is no creation without destruction, and it's the destruction of the false that makes way for re-creation. Short of that, you'll never become what you wish to be, or what you could be with me."

For the remainder of the drive, I hold the question of how to open his heart without weakening or undermining him, and listen for a reply. I hear nothing. Against my will, my heart hands down a verdict. Slowly and reluctantly, I accept it. I cannot open Randall's heart for him. Randall, and only Randall, can do that safely, if he wills it.

When Randall pulls his car into the driveway, my throat

swells. I go in silence to my chamber and find my suitcase. I open it on the bed and throw my things in a heap in the middle. I shake it down. I don't have the nerve to leave carefully and methodically. I close the case with a snap and turn to the door, and then remember my art. I open the case again and gather my dioramas from around the room. Randall comes and gently places his hands on my arms.

"Don't do this, Colette, don't run away. Not now."

With all the force of my will, I hold back tears and shake my head. "I'm not running away. I'm accepting that we're not good for each other now."

"I know we haven't had sex often enough. I can change that."

"A few weeks ago, I started practicing tantra on my own. It's been far more satisfying than the kind of sex we've been having on the couch."

Randall opens his mouth. His eyes grow red as if tears are near. He clears his throat and asks, "What are these boxes?"

"My dioramas."

"Show them to me?"

I struggle with my reluctance. He was never curious before. "I didn't before because you never asked."

"You never said."

"I did. Often." I relent and open my favorite. I may as well show him. His opinion no longer matters and his support was never mine to lose. I take the largest box to the altar and open it on its hinges. After a long pause, he comes and sits next to me. Pain stains my heart. This is the first time he has sat on the cushion that we chose for him.

Randall explores the box, running his fingers over the fine grain of the mahogany exterior, and the glass windows that cover each half of the box that stands open like a book. He gazes at the sequences of composited flats that make up the three-dimensional construct and says wistfully, "Each is like an opera set, or a pop-up theater for kids. But the one on the left is distorted. Disturbing. I thought you didn't like that."

I talk him through it. "Each depicts the landscape you can see from the rose garden at Yarra Spur. The one on the left shows what I see there, and the one on the right shows what's there." I turn the open book around so that we can see its covers. "The realistic one is based on a photo. The table engraved here shows the elements with their actual areas." I point to the table behind the proportionate model. "The disproportionate one is based on what I liked to look at. It shows the elements by the proportion of time I spent looking at them in the course of an hour on my favorite bench. Do you see? It shows how my likes and dislikes alter my perceptions."

Randall gasps in recognition. He says, "It's like a homunculus. It's brilliant. The solution is objectivity."

"It isn't a problem, it makes a point. One reflects the subjective and one the objective. Both are essential. But what's a homunculus?"

"On the cerebral cortex there's a map of the body's neurons. It's quite distorted. We are not uniformly innervated—for example, our senses are focused in our palms, eyes, and so on."

"You've lost sight of the subjective inner life. Which is the reason that I have to go now," I say, my voice breaking.

I stand resolutely and resume my careful packing.

He says with belated concern, "They may break. Leave them here, or let me send them to you."

I shake my head and push past him, heading for the front door, pulling my squeaking suitcase, which sounds like unkind laughter at my failure to lead us out of the cul-de-sac of our precarious experiment. I turn back to say, "I want nothing more than to be your consort, but if I stay, my love for you will die, and we'll lose our chance forever."

"If you leave, it's over."

I smile incredulously and grunt in exasperation. "That's up to you. Don't you see? I'm nothing in the distorted diorama of your life. You can't have what you disregard. You turn it into nothing."

9

Moving On

I am sitting on the cottage floor painting an echidna that will peek out at toddlers from beneath the bathroom sink. I am enjoying the renovation work and taking a page from Randall's playbook—working as much as possible so as not to grieve. So far, Andy and I have torn out one Yarra Spur cottage and redone three of the five that remain. The décor was set by Reggie's grandma, who died several months ago and left an attic filled with a century's accumulation of household items; we used them to create an atmosphere of antique elegance. We aim now to appeal to multi-generational families, with antiques and walking trails for grandparents; food and wine and babysitting for parents; and for children, paintings of animal families and communities plus an adventure playground with ropes course and flying fox. The work is no substitute for a consort; I am not happy, but I am deeply content to leave behind the big city life of money and motion for one of character and creative action.

Absorbed in my work completing the final echidna, I barely notice the high-pitched squeak that signals that a truck is braking outside. I remain oblivious until the door bangs open and Andy rushes in, saying, "Drop that and run!"

I sit frozen in astonishment. "Is there a fire?"

"I'll tell you in the truck," he says impatiently.

When the outer door slams shut behind us, I stop in shock.

The winery truck is parked outside. The end of Reggie's sofa bed is visible beneath the tarp tied onto the back. Reggie is sitting impassively in her car, which is idling behind the truck. We must be leaving Yarra Spur, now and for good.

Andy jumps into the driver's seat and shouts, "Get in! Get in!"

I grab the heavy door, yank it open, and climb awkwardly into the passenger seat as he speeds away. I have just managed to close the dented door when we pass the white farmhouse and Oliver Wheeler's car races around us, stopping across the road to block our exit. He climbs out and hurries hippo-like toward the snub nose of our truck. When he reaches the grille, he lifts his face. It is a flushed blot criscrossed by a web of broken veins.

Oliver Wheeler raises his fists, pounds the hood, and shouts at Andy, "This truck is my property! You can't take it!"

Andy rolls down his window and shouts back, "I'll return it tomorrow."

"You don't have my permission to leave with that twat!"

Andy grabs the window frame and pushes his head and body out so far that he is barely balanced, and then fires his rage. "I quit!"

"You can't! You didn't give notice. Don't you bloody well forget who's boss! This place is mine!"

"Don't you bloody well forget what I know about you, Wheeler! If you make trouble for anyone, including the Greenes, I'll dob you in for your illegal sewerage outlet, and show the Metcalfs your water diversion, and word up Marilyn about your punting with the petty cash! You went too far this time, Wheeler, you shithouse yobbo!"

Oliver Wheeler slumps as if struck in the stomach. He turns and lumbers back to his car, crawls in, and lets it roll backward out of the way. Marilyn, who has returned from giving a tour, is standing with a line of customers at the front entrance to the tasting room. She looks unhappy, but unsurprised. The guests seem disappointed at the sudden resolution of this dramatic discord. When the road is clear, we resume our speedy exit. As Andy salutes the crowd sardonically, Yarra Spur disappears behind us and into our shared past. At the end of the driveway, he turns toward Melbourne. Reggie follows in the car.

As we pass Domaine Chandon, Andy glances over at me and frowns. I expect him to let off steam by teasing me roughly, but he says, "Good thing you're here. Reg and I need you now."

"What happened?"

"The Greenes were about to sell their vineyard to Reg when Wheeler got wind of it, and that's when the worm hit the ceiling. He threatened them, and Reg, and me, and that was it. She'd had it. So we loaded the truck and left."

"Did you expect to quit?"

"I've been fed up with that bloody idiot since I met him. If he'd kept shut, she'd have bought the Greene place, and managed the transition, and sold him grapes at a great price. It would have been a win-win-win, everybody happy. But the old bugger doesn't think, he only wants his way."

"What will happen to Yarra Spur?"

"He'll make cheap wine and go out of business."

If there is anything that I learned from Randall, it is how to shut down my emotions. But after we have gone several miles, and the shock wears off, and I have let disbelief and anger come and go, I begin to miss the paints and brushes that I left behind and to fixate on the bodiless echidna that will never be finished. I begin to cry.

Andy says, "If it's Denton you're worried about, you needn't. Gyorgos is keen to have you back. It seems he's worse than

185

Grandma for driving kitchen help away, and word down the pub is everyone's decided that last year's debacle was all Yan's fault."

"He wants me back?"

"I'd say so, I'd say so."

"I'm glad, but that's not it."

"Ah, right."

"It's—who's going to finish the echidna?" I am blubbering now, my top lip gooey, my sob-laugh catching in my throat. "I want my brushes."

Andy raises an eyebrow. "You've been hiding out in the cottages to be with the imaginary animals. It couldn't be something to do with the good doctor?"

I shrug and take a deep sigh and make a point of counting the gum trees as they whiz by. I change the subject. "Where is Lisa? And the baby?"

"Visiting Denton. Lisa can help with publicity for The Inn, which is a hotter project."

"And Ruth?"

"Glad you brought that up. When you told her she didn't know the difference between sacred and profane sex, she went to see the priest and he agreed. Turns out the Orthodox are not terribly ascetic. Makes you wonder about their sex life, doesn't it?"

I laugh. "No! I don't want to know!"

"Right, well, you and Ruth ought to see eye-to-eye now."

Andy's hands clench the jolting steering wheel as we hit a bump in the road, and bounce wildly along on the squeaking chassis. "We're like the Joads in this bucket of bolts."

"Andy! You've read *The Grapes of Wrath!* You never cease to amaze me."

Andy grins. "Ah, yeah, I've read a few books about grapes. And a few about the Macedon Ranges. Have you read the one about Hanging Rock?"

"No. What's Hanging Rock?"

"It's a rock formation near the Denton place. Some girls went missing there years ago, and trackers couldn't find 'em. Peter Weir made a film about it."

I laugh, and then gasp. It's like that painting at the National Gallery, the one called *Lost*. "Good thing we've got a born leader with us. We won't need tracking"

"Right-o, mate."

I summon my sense of adventure. I tell myself to feel loose and fancy-free, and to seize the day, but faced with impermanence, my body becomes a blob. My heart and my gut reject the constancy of change. I cycle silently through resignation, fear, sorrow, and denial, all the way through the snarling traffic of the sluggish streets of Melbourne. Finally, Andy and I begin to enjoy our ephemeral freedom, and to talk of our favorite spots in the city, the ones we would visit if we were backpackers visiting from Europe and the States. Finally, I sigh deeply. My mind draws a deadline in the sands of time, and resolves that by the end of this week, my body will have adjusted to this new reality, and my mind will have formed a new story at least as resilient as the old one.

As we clear the city, we see fallow fields that form a rich palette of blacks and browns. Near a range of low and rugged hills signaling the Dividing Range, as Andy and I are sharing stories of past moves, he turns the truck onto a road that heads up and east into the bush of Mount Macedon. As we climb, we pass conventions of sulfur-crested cockatoos, a lone koala chewing leaves in a gum tree, and cylinders of hay sitting fat and ready to nourish livestock.

"It feels a bit like coming home," I say.

"I could do with a little horse riding."

Miles on, while we are skirting golden sandstone walls, some of them graced by formal gates and hand-scripted signs, we glimpse between lines of trees stately houses and stud farms like Denton. The whole region appears to pre-date federation, when Victoria joined with other states. We seem to be moving both forward and back in time, as if slipping out of sync.

"I could have helped pack."

"Ay?"

"I was just painting. I could have helped you and Reg."

"Ah, yeah. Reg was afraid of what Wheeler would do. She wanted to keep you out of sight."

"When did you two know that we were leaving?"

"She must have known last night. The boot of the car was full."

"Hard to tell. She's always ready to travel."

"I still can't believe I left the bottling apparatus in the middle of a run."

"Is Reg hard hit?"

"She was wanking on about non-attachment, which means she'll be sooking for weeks."

"I can't take it in."

"Don't. We won't be here long."

"I have that feeling too."

"It isn't a feeling, it's a plan. Reg is going to train Melanie to care for the vines and wines, Lisa and I are going to research places to set up a retreat center with fine wines and cuisine, and you're going to teach Gyorgos to make decent crêpes and croissants."

"You've been thinking about this for a while!"

"Almost a year now."

"Since the Cup Carnival?"

"Right in one. She'll be apples, mate, she'll be apples."

"Why can't she be grapes?" I have the sense of the world spinning, as if the curves in the road were setting us on a dance of forgetting.

"That's like asking why Matilda waltzed. You'll never make an Aussie."

"Then you and Reg'll have to take us someplace else. Be sure to use your world map when you're scheming."

Andy smiles slyly, and gives me a wink.

10
Tree of Life

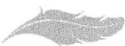

This year we spend our Cup Carnival week safely away from Denton at Anne's beach house near Blairgowire. Here we can enjoy the wild waters of the Southern Ocean and the tranquil waters of Port Philip Bay, and our first gathering as a separate community. Andy and Lisa, Reg and Graeme, and I have been discussing our shared future—especially the retreat center that will define our fertile contribution to the social evolution of our species, and through that to the survival of what Melissa is calling the nested bodies of humanity, of habitats, and of the body of life. It is a heady but grounded time, and for me a chance to harken back to, and move forward from, the spiritual awakening through sexuality that began on the ocean beach.

The visit is about to culminate with a fancy dress party to which we have invited Ronnie, Liz, and Reggie's Uni friends, who will dine with us and then party-hop on to Portsea. To honor the spirit of the Pacific Rim, I am preparing Tasmanian salmon from Macquarie Harbour, where barometric tides flow cold and fast, and farmed fish struggle in pristine currents and thrive as in the waters of Alaska. With that we will serve kiwi and qandong with apple for freshness; a baked timbale of New World potatoes with bush tomatoes and African red pepper for fire; and glasses of lightly oaked California chardonnay for innovation.

The fancy dress theme is two-fer—each couple coming in one

costume. Liz and Ronnie arrive first and use a back bedroom to style their costume, which they are calling "harmonic convergence." I guess from their hints that they will soon emerge looking like a two-headed Greek Goddess in one toga, each holding a harmonica in the free hand. Louis and Emily arrive and join the group, which is gathering around the barbeque. I look up from the grill to see them dressed as a horse with two heads, one at each end. They run back and forth and prance sideways in a comical mock-dressage, and ask people to guess what they are.

"Janus horse," I say without hesitation. "We've been looking to the past and future all week, and thinking of the old Roman Janus heads." Then—and with each correct guess that follows—we toast visual tropes. Hal and Dutchy arrive with the baby. Hal is a Roman soldier, Spartacus style; Dutchy is dressed in a black wig and tight leopard-print dress and holding a bagel in one hand; and Jos is swaddled in a towel. When Jos smiles beatifically, the group's silence hovers between bafflement and shock, and Emily says tentatively, "The Holy Family?"

"Yes!" Hal says with a smile. "Yeshua—called Jesus by the Greeks—was probably a child of rape by a Roman soldier called Flavius!" When the silence dilates, he asks, "Too much?"

"To too much!" Ronnie says, and we all toast Emily quietly.

Clive and Laura come as the people in the American Gothic painting by Whistler, holding a large frame that completes the picture; Rog and Judy come as a black cockatoo, each as a wing with the body suspended in between, their movements choreographed to evoke flight; Andy and Lisa and the baby as three crests of one large wave that is made of what appears to be singed canvas salvaged from last year's tent fire; and Graeme and Reg as vine leaves trying to cover a cluster of wild grapes.

I say, "And I come as a chef!" I lift a platter laden with

parchment wrapped salmon and lead the way indoors to the already set row of tables that has displaced the furniture in the living and dining area. I am pleased to see—when we are all seated, and Reg has toasted constant friends—that everyone has found something on the table to enjoy, and that they seem increasingly content as Reg and Graeme turn the conversation to their third. Graeme reads in his deep, resonant voice a poem by Rumi Through Barks, "Their two spirits go out from them as one. Whenever two are linked this way another comes from the unseen," and so on. After that Reg asks everyone to close their eyes and visualize being on their death beds, and to think for a time of what they want to have done as a life work that will make the world a better place, that is, of the third that they would like to create together.

When the guests have mentioned paid work, and blood families and good times, I see that they are not engaged. They have not thought about it, and are not in the mood for a contemplative party game. Perhaps sensing our disappointment, Dutchy asks, while spooning timbale into Jos' eager mouth, "Tell us about your thirds?"

Andy and Lisa look at each other. Lisa looks at Reg, who says, "Graeme and I want to develop ways to relate to changes in time and place in real time, and to help connect people to the full scope of their fertile possibilities so that they can discern the next step—and the next, and the next—toward the lives they want to create and the legacies they want to leave behind."

"And how will you assess all of that?"

"We won't," Graeme smiles.

"Experience that hones intuition," Reg says.

"And you, Andy and Lisa?" Dutchy asks.

All eyes turn to Andy now. He looks at Lisa, who nods.

"We have our child, and we'd like to adopt a habitat. One that's been neglected and abused and that needs protection and care and tending. With time we'll develop it into an Eden land—a habitat that can sustain itself indefinitely, and that our community can live in and with."

There is a stunned silence that Hal breaks, saying, "Not what I expected from you, Andy!"

"You never said," Judy adds diplomatically.

"You never asked," Andy replies. "You can only dole out pesticides for so long without noticing that it's probably a bad idea. You're drinking them right now."

"Thanks for that," Laura says.

"No worries," Andy replies ironically.

"And you?" Clive asks, looking at me.

"I want to use art to explore fertility, and to help others—especially women—explore what it is and means now, in the age of birth control."

"And who'll be paying for all the castles in the sky? Your grandma?" Rog asks Reg with a sardonic smile.

"We will. We'll be buying some land and setting up a fertility retreat center."

"You'll need some capital," Rog persists.

"We're looking for investors and lenders."

"It's good to know that you have a plan," Louis says.

"And imagination," Laura says.

"Good luck with all that," Rog says. "Now can we play cards?"

"You don't want to dance?" Clive asks.

"Too many toasts," Rog replies.

At eleven o'clock, after light conversation and games and a shared dramatic reading of a passage from a novel about the famous racehorse Phar Lap, Reg's University friends leave for other parties, and Liz and Ronnie change back into their street clothes and bid Reg a tearful goodbye.

"Tired and emotional?" I ask Reg, using the tabloid euphemism for drunk.

"I've told them I may not see them again before we go."

We had not talked of leaving soon. "That makes it all very immediate."

As we clean up inside and out, there is a loud knock at the door. A tall figure, presumably a man, enters. I am a little frightened by his costume, a leather poncho and bucket-like helmet with horizontal eye slits.

"It's Ned Kelly!" says Andy. "And in full battle armor."

"Welcome, Ned," says Lisa.

"Who?" I try to see into the slits but see only glints of white.

"You haven't been to the Melbourne Gaol, I see," says Dutchy. "Ned Kelly iss the most famous bush ranger in the hisstory of Victoria. This iss his armor."

"He was an outlaw," says Graeme.

They are having me on. This is a new game. "Am I supposed to guess?"

The apparition tips forward and backward to indicate yes.

"Sean?"

The apparition swivels back and forth to indicate no.

"Geoff?"

More swiveling.

"Yan?"

The apparition reaches up and removes its helmet.

For a full minute, I am too shocked and confused to respond, and then I am catapulted from misery to joy. *He chose me! He chose us!* I forget heartbreak and worry and delve into the delicious dizziness of this reunion with lost love. Randall sheds the body armor. His anxious expression and tense shoulders are holding an uneasy mix of love and fear. I run to him and throw my arms around his shoulders. For many long moments, I am aware of nothing other than his breathing, his heartbeat, and the feeling of his belly opening to mine.

Randall's body feels wonderful, and strange. I had forgotten the hair on the back of his fingers, the curve of his pelvis, the bony line of his spine, and the wiry texture of his hair. I expected love and intimacy to make memory constant, to keep us in sync, but it takes many bright flashes of the present moment to erase the alterations in memory wrought by time, absence, and experience, to correct the vagaries of sense and perception, and to restore the immediacy of a fluid, living connection. Soon our breathing is alternating with regularity and his vitality is awakening mine. I memorize him now as best I can, taking a tactile hologram of him to carry in my body in case this is our only chance to deepen a living connection that may bind us together through time and timelessness.

After several minutes, I whisper shyly in his ear, "You feel different."

He grips my ribs in a tighter embrace. "Tell me I haven't lost you!"

I hear cars start and realize that the others have gone out, push his chest away and look deep into his eyes. The intensity of his gaze and my response are too much to bear. I lower my gaze. "I love you still. I always will."

Randall puts his hands behind my nape and presses his lips to my forehead. "I slept in your room every night after you left me! I can't believe I didn't do it before. I was awful to you! Can you forgive me?"

"You needn't be afraid. I'm here with you. I'm yours."

"Everything was closing in on me then. I didn't know if I could sustain the pressure."

"I should have been able to get through to you, to show you a way out. But I couldn't."

Randall snorts and says sharply, "Melissa said you felt like a pox doctor's tart."

I am glad that I cannot see Randall's pain as Graeme does. It is enough to feel, through him, his heavy weight of shock and sorrow. Fortunately my small poise is enough to hold us now as his heart opens to mine and mine to his. I put my arms around his shoulders, gather my strength, and reply, "I shouldn't have let you take it out on me then, and I won't let you do it now. You can't treat me that way again!"

"I wouldn't want to but I don't understand what happened. I'm too raw."

"We'll figure it out. Together. As equal partners." I lower my palms gently to rest on his back ribs and whisper, "Tell me what changed your mind."

Randall grunts. His voice catches. A wave of sorrow rises and passes. "When I told Stan about my parents he tried to love me as he had. He struggled to care for me and to continue as my mentor. But he couldn't. He was too angry. He felt I'd betrayed his trust. He felt I wasn't Jewish. And then he sat shiva for me in his heart as if I had died to him. That was when I missed you most. I wanted to hold you and to feel the blessing of you!"

We both know the harm that comes of secrets. "You're free of secrets now, and of the harm they can do."

"After that I told everyone, and found out who my friends are, who recognizes me as a Jew who both wrestles God and crosses boundaries."

"What you are is up to you and no one else. Which is the

reason that I need to know that you know and can tell me."

"I didn't before I put it on you," he confesses. "I thought the world of Stan. When he and Ellie were against you, I blamed you for that, and when they cut me off I blamed you for that, too. I'm sorry! I'm so ashamed!"

"No, no. Don't punish yourself, or me. Trust that we can love and forgive ourselves and Stan and Ellie."

Randall's breathing eases. He sighs deeply. His shoulders relax. "Everything's come apart."

"Everything's coming together. You faced your fears. You acknowledged the meaning of our lives. That gives us the chance to realize our dreams."

"Help me move on?" Randall blurts in a strained voice.

"Yes! But how long do we have? When do you have to go back?"

"I don't. I closed on the condo and sold my practice to David and Stan."

I push his chest and look wildly into his eyes. "You left your practice?"

"I want to do a new kind of fertility work, with you, and for you. I want to live openly and freely with you and with the people who matter to you. To us."

I close my eyes and press his hand to my lips. No vessel of words or ideas, no container made or unmade could hold the fullness of our unborn future. "You're becoming the man I fell in love with."

"I tried to be like Maimonides but I didn't go far enough. He was a master of aphrodisiacs. He worked with fertility, not infertility. I want to do that. I want to intervene early and gently, to support rather than undermine the erotic bond, to make the bedroom a place for blissful union rather than a workplace or a battleground. I want to join my scientific fertility to your artistic creativity."

I take his hands and look into his eyes. "That's a wonderful vision. I want to give birth to that with you now and until I'm lying on my death bed."

Randall's body is shaking. His radical departure from the past is extraordinarily brave, an act of destruction and creation that requires everything he has and is and can become.

I continue in a voice of comfort, "You're talking of more than fertility. You're talking of continuation that's conscious, loving, creative, and hopeful."

When he speaks again, it is with a slight accent and a tone that is touched by tears. "It's the ongoing evolution of the tree of life in all its tangible and intangible manifestations."

Something in his voice enters into my ears and flows down my spine to my root. Something new is arising that has the weight of the eternal and the lightness of the new. "You're different than you were, but still unformed, still raw."

"I have no words for it, but I do have a new practice to share with you."

"Now?"

"Now."

I go to turn up the heat and return to take his hand and lead him to the back bedroom where we undress each other with fumbling, breathless urgency. He chases me into the bathroom where we wash each other with playful excitement. Then we return to the bed and dry each other lightly.

We sit face to face, my legs wrapped around his hips. We gaze at each other until the veils within, which are made of cares and habits, grow thin. When we are relaxed, and have felt our energy sink below our navels, we become aware of energy gathering between our bodies.

"Our third," I whisper.

Randall begins quietly intoning selected verses of the Song of Songs, first in Hebrew and then in English. I don't know the verses of response, so he sings those as well, and then says,

"Through us, the masculine aspects of the One joins its feminine aspects."

Randall puts his left arm around my back and pulls me close until our foreheads touch. He brings his right hand between our breastbones with the thumb side resting against his and the little finger side resting against mine. I encircle his back with my left arm and press my palm against his. We close our eyes and sit in silence for a full minute. I feel him sinking into *a* state of peace. After a time of silent communication, he laughs deep in his throat and whispers. "Just for you, a custom visualization of the Jewish tree of life, *on peut dire c'est l'arbre de la vie Celtique et Hindou.*"

"I forgot that you were a doctor rabbi comedian."

"*HaShem* is laughing. His breath is ruffling the trees outside."

Randall takes a deep breath and I open my eyes to the beauty of his joyful face and let my eyelids close again, and my ears drink in his words.

"We'll start at the places where our bodies rest on our marriage bed, at *malkhut*, where the two worlds meet. Hidden in *malkhut* is a tiny seed of spirit, smaller than an acorn, able to grow high enough to shelter the angels, and the archangels. Breathe in the spring air where buds will soon burst, breathe out to nourish the seed of spirit … breathe in, breathe out … see the seed of spirit send a root far down into the earth to draw her sustenance … see the root and its growing shoot expel waste into the earth to feed the living soil … "

Randall's voice and energy steady us. I visualize our spirit seed retreating into potentiality, sending roots down toward the earth below, and shoots up into our bodies above.

"I see it!"

Randall slides his palms down my back and spreads his fingers so that they touch the middle of my sacrum. His voice falls like a gently cascading stream as he says, "Let your energy sink low, and lower, flowing from the vault above your skull into the cup below your pelvis... allow the energy that comes down to us from the heavens to flow with it." After a pause, Randall slides his palms down until his fingers reach the tip of my tailbone, and then down to and under the edge of the muscles that sling between my pubis and tailbone, and suspend the flesh between my thighs. His voice cascades downward again as he says, "And now let your energy fall all the way to the surface beneath you."

I let the energy of my being stream toward my spine and down along the front of my spine like the headwaters of a stream that flows down from the heavens, through my body, and into the earth. Gradually, the midpoint of my energy descends until it is resting behind my yoni, and touching Randall's. As our energies become confluent, they fill the space between our roots with dark warmth and a pool of light.

"I feel it, and see it!"

Randall takes a full breath and continues, "Now feel our seed push up transparent, luminescent shoots, one into your root and one into mine ... see your body shrink to the size of a pea and rest on the tip of the shoot as it rises steadily up to form the trunk of your growing tree of life ... see the shoot filling the soul's lamp with the blue light of consciousness ... feel the delicate and intangible trunk of the tree of life lifting your tiny body ... ascend through the central channel of your subtle body all the way through the secret chakra in the pelvis and up to *yesod*, where you rest, and where the tree sends out branches…"

After an interval, I see and feel what he is describing. "I feel it! I feel it in you, and feel it mirrored in me."

Randall guides our energy outward from the central axis along the branches to *hod*, which he links to assertion, and to *netzach*, which he links to receptivity, and then returns to the center to rest at *yesod*, the point of harmony, where *hod* and *netzach* are in balance. He guides us up through the sun center to *tiferet*, the lower heart center, where he follows branches to *gevurah*, or restraint, and *chesed*, or reckless love, and then returns to the center at *tiferet*, the fulcrum of compassion, the place where *gevurah* and *chesed* join in strength and rest in balance. He guides us upward then to the *point vierge*, the upper heart center which with the lower center forms the *nous*, the eye of the heart, the seat of beauty that perceives and receives sweet divine love and returns it with steadfast joy.

I realize that I am breathing in as he breathes out. "I feel it! Mmmm. Thank you for bringing us here, and for holding us here. This must be heaven."

I hear Randall laugh deep in his throat and then continue, "Now we rest in sacred union on the tip of the trunk as it rises up through the throat chakra like the white drop … and higher, ever higher, beyond the subtle body, beyond the lamp of the *ruach* and the *neshama*, into *chayah*, the ethereal body, where the lamps of our souls can touch the light of the realms of higher consciousnes."

I exhale sharply in the briefest of laughs. "No higher?"

"Patience," he whispers fondly. "We rest in *chayah*, the realm from which thoughts arise, where the translucent, luminous trunk of the tree of life sends branches out to form, or *chochma*, and to essence, or *binah*, and we rest in the center at *daat*, the balance of knowing where *chochma* and *binah* meet…"

My being fills with joy to the point of our awareness. The joy may be his, or may be mine through his being, and the words that express his Judaic path to awakening.

"We rest on the trunk at *daat* while the tip of the shoot continues to rise above us into the highest body of the soul, the *Yehidah*, where duality dissolves … we cannot enter this realm, from which intentions arise, except in the highest of altered states … and so we rest below that realm of unity and look up at the crown of the tree of life, and sense the presence of *keter* in awe, and see in it the oak of wisdom of the Druids, and the top of Yggdrasil, the Vikings' world tree… we look in wonder at this unborn reality, and ask to accept what it is given to us to know of the realm of unity beyond human understanding …"

The boundaries between us and between the tangible and intangible worlds seem to dissolve as our bodies unite and align with heaven and earth. My awareness fills with white, exalting light.

"Now, we look down, away from *keter*, and descend along the trunk of the tree from *daat*, knowledge… to the flame of the lamp that burns above the crown … and follow the translucent trunk through the delicate channel of the lamp, descending like the red drop through the central channel … resting in *tiferet* with beauty and compassion and then in *yesod* with harmony and then in *malkhut*, the root, where the inner and outer worlds meet, where we join the sovereignty of our bodies, *nefesh* with *nefesh*, inviting the grace of *HaShem*."

Randall lifts my yoni onto his lingam, which is so hard that we join uncomfortably. I lean forward, rest my belly against his, and hold his gaze. Our energy joins now at all levels, and rises above our crowns. The kundalini energy rises from our joined roots in a spiral of fire that we feed with our breath and that tingles upward and outward in waves. I can tell by Randall's face that he feels it too. His expression metamorphoses from disbelief to wonder to joy to love to ecstasy. He climaxes rapidly.

I realize after a minute, that he has not ejaculated. When the wave of energy ebbs, and we come to rest, he says, panting, "The *kundalini* snakes coiled around our trees of life!"

"Yes! We must be in the Garden! One with each other and with—with—"

"The One life joined by the One love!" After a moment his face falls. "The end of our joining will be like another fall. How will we bear it?"

I laugh giddily. "We are here now, together, and can relive it whenever we remember it."

After a pause, his expression of joy returns. "We can return to it together, and apart."

"How did you learn to orgasm without ejaculation?"

"Graeme told me about acupressure points."

Randall's body separates from mine. He is right; the end is like a loss. I try to sustain our joy with the memory of ecstasy. Randall pulls me gently down onto the bed and lies on top of me. The delicious touch of his soft penis raises a frisson of pleasure that flows, and then ebbs into profound bliss. He guides his soft lingam into my yoni. A valley orgasm rises and spreads up my back to my crown. Randall's lingam grows hard, and he moves slowly and shallowly, extending my valley before moving deeply and quickly and propelling us both to an intense, full-body peak. Again, he does not ejaculate.

"I want to pleasure you," I say. I suck his lower lip, and then add, "Tell me what you want."

"To give you Graeme's second gift."

"His second gift?"

"Lie down."

Randall gives me a long, sensual massage of efflurages and palming that climaxes in a massage of my yoni. He brings me to another intense peak, from which I return to a high valley. He kneels upright on the floor and pulls my hips up to join with him again. We hold an ecstasy that seems inclusive of every possible emotion and each conceivable state of being. Randall holds this state, rocking slowly and gently for a long time until we dissolve all boundaries. Then he releases his sacred fluid.

He drops down on the bed and lies with me. I feel the memory of shared joy imprinted in our beings, and in the beings of those connected to us by love. In this state, I can transform the bitterest memories of samsara by mixing them with the sweet nectar of our nirvana. We lie on the pillows, full in every way, until our heart light shines out to illuminate our sleep.

Epilogue

Melissa and I and her friend Consuela exit the main entrance of the lodge building of the Saltspring Fertility Center and walk north, through the playground and west on a rising trail to a scenic overlook where the trunks of first growth Douglas fir, hemlock and red and yellow cedar trees give way to a rocky outcropping.

"This part of Saltspring Island is a provincial park," I say, hopping up to the highest stretch of granite. "That's Vancouver Island—and Cow, or Cowichan Bay."

"Beautiful!" Melissa says. "How did you get land next to this park?"

"Randall had a patient who inherited this land from his family. They were loggers. When we got here ten years ago there was a ban on logging and so Randall was able to persuade him that we could make good use of the land, and that he should lease it to us. He loves it here—he sails with Reg, and eats my French cuisine—mostly against Randall's advice, and takes our classes. He gave us a 99-year lease a few years ago, and then formed a board and a trust that forgave our loans. So the land is secure, and we're under no pressure to profit."

"That's lucky," Consuela says. "If you like it here. It's so dense and green it must rain all the time."

I laugh. "We do meditate a lot in the winter dark."

We move to another point from which we enjoy a sweeping view of the fields in the bottomlands below, of Fulford Harbor and its ferry, the Gulf and San Juan Islands nearby, and the lower B.C. mainland in the distance.

"The habitat looks healthy!" says Melissa.

"It was all clear-cut at one point, and it's recovering well but still far from mature. On our land we have first, second and third growth and recent clear cut and we're restoring it as we try habitat integration and enhancement."

"Meaning what?" Asks Consuela.

"We're building tree houses and cob houses in forest that we're restoring, and seeding mushrooms and indigenous berries, and trying a little controlled burning. We're also looking at Sitk'sun and Nou-chah-nulth recipes and traditional methods of shellfish and seaweed farming."

"When does the session start?" Melissa asks with a frown.

"We have plenty of time before sunset, but let's start back now."

I lead them back into the twilight of the trail and down toward the lodge, turning and slowing to say, "I want to thank you for sharing your expertise and ideas. It's been difficult but essential."

"It's been flat-out depressing," Consuela says. "You guys and your habitat extinction, and Melissa with chronic poisoning of humans."

"And you and me with birth defects and autism and cancer and neurodegenerative diseases. What's left to face?" Melissa asks warily.

"Nothing we don't know, and everything we haven't felt and turned into action," I say.

Melissa sighs. "That'll be a relief—especially for the kids—and their guilty parents."

"Reg implied that anyone who's ever used a plastic bag has been part of the problem," Connie says.

"Which is basically true," Melissa says. "We're all at fault."

"Speak for yourself!"

"I am."

I point out the mushrooms and berries, and the places where the barn and pastures and hothouse will be—and, someday, we hope, the community school and fertility complex. We go around the lodge this time and then veer north from the back entrance to the forest theatre. It has a removable membrane roof that has been stowed below the stage on this fine day; seating for 200, and an outer ring of newly planted alders encircled by a water feature that divides and flows around the perimeter. Randall and Andy have had fun adding lighting and more multimedia than they need to augment the visualization that Reggie has prepared for us. We find her and ask if she needs anything. She shakes her head and smiles broadly.

"I've never had so much fuel for *tonglen*. I'm giddy!"

"What's that?" Melissa asks.

"Giving and talking, using the defilements in the surround to destroy personal ones."

"That works?" Consuela says skeptically.

"It takes practice. It's perfect for today. I don't want to let you down."

"Let us down?"

"You need this. We all do."

Melissa and Connie and I go to the back rows opposite the end of the proscenium stage that is surrounded on three sides by folding chairs on risers. Randall, Andy, Lisa, and Graeme join us, and the theater is soon full. Jilly and Tom, friends of Andy who have come to live with us, do the technical support which begins very simply with a spotlight trained on Reg, who is sitting center stage on my pad and cushion, meditating in half Lotus with her hands positioned in a beginner's *mudra*. The lights go up slowly on the membrane screen that encircles the theater with a high oval panorama comprised of images of pristine habitats. We hear Reggie's voice but her lips do not move. She pre-recorded it so that Jilly and Tom could synchronize her voice with sound and images. We also hear birdsong that corresponds with the habitats and that calls responses from the forest that spread outward like a wave.

"It is 1491 in North America. The white and grey tides are about to arrive bringing distant plagues and a ten-millenium-long habit of turning forest into field, and of spending the future of life on thoughtless consumption and destruction."

We hear the sounds of axes and saws felling trees, of mills turning trunks into planks, of sanders and drills. The sounds are soft but unmistakable, and merge into noise that obscures the birdsong.

"I will now read a list of dead and dying watersheds, with the percentage of the habitat destroyed by us between then and now."

Reggie's voice solemnly intones the first of the dead places in our hemisphere that were once home to life on which the biome—and thus the whole of our species—depended. We hear a clock ticking and voices chanting in time with Reggie and the clock. The sounds form an inexorable dirge as the images above us begin to darken from the midpoint behind center stage outward in both directions. The eastern hardwood forests fade to black, and those of Mississippia, and those of the west, and finally those of Cascadia, which dim but do not disappear into the dark of nothingness. When we can no longer see one another, Melissa grasps my hand and Consuela's and whispers a chant.

"No … no … no … no. … "

The sound cuts out. We hear crying. Reggie's voice begins again, "We have a choice between the modern course to death and destruction that began with the last ice age and continued with the white tide of colonialism," she says, speaking from the stage now, "and the restoration that may still be in our power to effect."

The spotlight rises. The images on the oval screen rise, beginning at the back and moving to the front. Melissa releases a sigh of relief and then calls out.

"Restoration!" Others take up the call, and soon we are all standing and chanting thunderously, "Restoration. Restoration. Restoration…" After a minute the audience breaks into applause; after another minute we resume our seats.

Reggie continues, "Now is your chance to commit to restoration by making a pledge in company with our community. Who will start?"

The first pledges—presumably from those members who have thought and done the least for the most—are simple, and come up, popcorn style, from the front rows of guests:

"I'm going to wear vintage clothing and buy vintage furniture."

"I'm going to take the bus—when I can."

"I'm going to shop at the farmer's market instead of the supermarket."

"I'm going to plant a garden."

"I'm going to bike to work."

"I'm going to walk instead of ride."

"I'm going to compost."

"I'm going to create a kinetic sculpture to power my outdoor lights."

"I'm going to plant flowers, shrubs and trees on my street."

"I'm going to reclaim materials from construction sites when I build my shed."

The pledges become more substantial.

"I'm going to buy an electric car and power it with solar panels."

"I'm going to capture rainwater for myself, and maybe with my neighbors."

"I'm a landscaper, and I'm going to spread bioswales."

"I'm a builder and I'm going to look for clients who want to cut energy use so that I can use more natural light and geothermal power in my projects."

"I'm going to distribute heirloom seeds that I got from my grandfather."

The popcorn slows. Those who have thought—or sought inspiration or competition—offer more substantial vows.

Doug says, "When I encounter a problem, instead of responding to it with an equal and opposite reaction, I will let it transform me the way a photon transforms an electron."

Reggie laughs and says, "We should consult you when we take on higher order transformations!"

Father Sean says, "Every time I remember to do it, I'm going to ask myself, how do I do the right thing, right now?"

"Very philosophical!" Melissa laughs.

"Good continuous practice," I say.

"It's no more or less than faith in practice," he says with a wink at Consuela.

An unfamiliar man with a shaggy black beard, pale eyes, and large silver ear studs stands and says, "I live up island off the grid on a fair piece of land. I make my living online, and earn enough to experiment. Right now I have my family in a small trailer while we build a low-impact, self-sufficient house. If I add satellite pods I'll be able to invite friends and creatives to come and stay and collaborate on creating local, sustainable businesses. If I do that, I can let them stay rent-free in exchange for habitat restoration."

Randall says, "Let us know how we can support that."

Reggie's mother, Anne, stands, folds her hands formally on the waist band of her tweed skirt, and says, "I'm a gardener, and I don't want to wait twenty years for my new organic methods to bring my soil up to par. I'm going to find a way to produce good soil. When I have all I need, I'll start selling it." Anne nods sharply and smiles. "I'll be delighted to be back in business."

Andy says, "We don't know how to live in community with the forest. When I finish up in fabro, I'm going to find a way to become a habitat integrator and a teacher of it."

Gyorgos stands and says with theatrical resignation, "I see foraging in my future. I've already switched the theme of Denton Inn to bush life, and I'll be kicking off my new menus with an innovative cuisine based on bush tucker. I'll start with bush tomatoes and basil, and invasive species like hare and feral pig, and then get onto Aboriginals who know the habitats and what's edible and what's not. I'll create a new palate for our region of Victoria." Gyorgos sits.

Ruth stands and says, "I'm going to volunteer to move the Greek Orthodox Church toward the living paradigm. I'll work with congregations to review their energy and water use, and to design landscaping and greening and other practices that align—and evolve—with our present understanding of faith in action."

An elderly woman stands and, struggling with her Scandinavian habit of avoiding personal attention, says, "I'm

Melissa's mother, and this is Colette's mother. We want to start a club that uses old fabric and fibers for knitting and quilting and embroidery projects. I'm tired of throwing good material away."

Pea stands and says, "I want to found a day care home that incorporates preventive pediatrics in early childhood education, and when that succeeds, to found a network of similar homes. Self-care begins at birth—and before—and we miss our chance to support that by teaching it late—or not at all."

Pippy pipes up, "We could build a detached structure and power it with solar."

Pea sits and blows Pippy a kiss. A man with a long maple beard and long hair stands. He is wearing open sandals covered in mud. He says, "I already took my old solar panels to the landfill and put them next to the old televisions. I've put a new cob floor in my workshop and piped hot spring water through it. If that works, I'll heat my house the same way."

"A hundred bucks says you can't do it," teases Doug.

The man laughs as he sits. "You're on. I'll take it now."

"I'll bring it when you finish."

A young man with an Aussie accent stands and says, "I'm going to design storm shutters that regulate heat and moisture in all weather. I'm going to try to press bark to make shells, spray in recycled fiber insulation, and surround them with denim baffles. I'll lock them from the inside. When I'm done with them nothing will get in around them or through them!"

A small claque of young men seated by Andy whoops and cheers. The young man bows comically to his team before sitting down.

Sarah stands and says tremulously, "I'm going to move here and join your community and teach yoga to you and your retreatants and students. I've been sitting for some time with the realization that we can't all have children. I feel blessed now to know that we can all be fertile."

Randall says, "I was hoping that you and Doug and Melissa and John would all come here to live—and bring your partners and families with you."

John stands and says, "I plan to continue working at the clinic that I founded based on my work with Melissa. Our small groups practice habitat restoration as part of our year-long course in medical wisdom yoga. We've bought or controlled enough property at the top of a small watershed to create a pesticide- and herbicide-free area around a stream where we'll be able to start residential habitat restoration."

My brother Sean stands and says, "I want to work with John to create a new musical instrument to take into the wild to catalyze spontaneous restoration. The idea will be to express the body's healing response to the body of life and turn it into a soundscape that revives player and listener and habitat as one."

John asks, "Analog?"

"Analog and digital."

John says gamely, "Let's do it."

Melanie says, "I want to move to the Olympic Peninsula and start a sheep to shawl competition that draws people from the islands and spreads the sustainable raising of sheep and goats— and at the same time encourages the development of minimally modified agricultural environments."

Lisa stands and says firmly, "I'm going to become a developer. The idea would be to develop eco-villages dedicated to habitat restoration. If capital can't do it, I'll turn to cooperative models."

Melissa stands and says, "I want to found a medical clinic that develops the emerging paradigm. I would begin with a patient-led team of a family practitioner, hands on healer, counselor, and habitat restorer. We'd support patients in being and becoming care and cure, and reversing causes of illness. The paradigm should become richer and richer in meaning as we restore the body of life. I'll research places when I leave."

Reggie stands. Her countenance becomes luminous. "All rise and join me in sharing a last round of applause with everyone who has made or witnessed a vow." The audience applauds again.

After a few minutes Reggie signals silence and says, "We who have founded this community are grateful that you have joined us in our metamorphosis and shared with us your unique gifts of life. We will leave you now with seven words to contemplate as you consider your next moves.

"The first word is extensive, which refers to new cosmologies that unite life in time with the protean universe;

"The second word is dynamic, which reminds us that matter and energy are fluid, changing, fluctuating, and yet orderly with respect to time;

'The third word is generative, which expresses the constant transformation of matter and energy through destructive creation and creative destruction;

"The fourth word is sacred, which conveys our direct, devotional connection with the One Life in space and time;

"The fifth word is clean, by which we refer to the state in which life takes in what nourishes it and puts out what doesn't;

"The sixth word is fertile, which is the full expression of the One Life in all its forms, and of each life that begins and continues until it transforms;

"The seventh word is cure, by which we refer to the end and reconciliation of destructive processes and the initiation of creative ones. May you become love and faith and thrive in action for life."

Melissa, Consuela and I stand and move out toward the pasture, motioning to our partners to join us. When Randall reaches us he darts toward Consuela and shakes her hand, "Good to see you," and then embraces Melissa warmly. "We're using your work, Connie, in our teaching of cause and effect, and yours, Missy, in our teachings on the body and the minimization of chronic poisoning. Our curriculum wouldn't be half what it has become without you."

"That's my Connie," Pippy says proudly.

Seeing Dan's wary expression I say, "And that's my BFF, Melissa—and Reggie and Lisa and Connie. Group hug!" I reach out and embrace the women—and their men—who gave birth to the thirds and group spirits that are holding our community, and offer a silent prayer for union and harmony.

Acknowledgments

For a deepening understanding of biological time in eternity, of the full extent of the human body, and of its interface with the bodies of species, habitats, and life on Earth, I send love and gratitude to the multifaith communities of Seattle and Melbourne and itinerant teachers of faith and practice. Those who did most to lead me beyond the bounds of modern medicine and modernity to a world of ideas and methods for care and cure, and to lead me beyond a puzzled reading of metamorphosis in Ovid and Shakespeare to living and embodying transformation, I offer deep gratitude to: Silversong Belcourt, Cynthia Bourgeault, Geshe Doga, Ted Falcon, Matthew Fox, Phil Gerson, Thomas Keneally, Gen Khedrup, Kathy Kizilos, Rich Lang, Lora-Ellen McKinney, Philip Maisel, Daniel Matt, Harrison Moretz, Weldon Nisly, Jamal Rachman, Jon Ramer, Reggie Ray, Craig Rennebohm, Phabongkha Rinpoche, Ari Roth, Zalman Schachter-Shalomi, Rami Shapiro, Rodney Smith, Jan Watson, the Campion Center, La Casa Maria, Christian Peacemaker Teams, the Compassionate Action Network, Earth Ministries, the Melbourne Holocaust Museum, Naropa University, the Nordic Heritage Center, Sakya Monastery, and Seattle Yoga Arts.

In the interests of including those who are distant in time and place, and whose words allow personal, embodied psychosocial evolution through their books, I express undying gratitude to:

Adam Frank, Arthur Eddington, Aldous Huxley, the authors of *Real Collaboration: What it Takes for Global Health to Succeed*, Arthur Green, Marc Oaknin, Lynn Bauman, Mantak Chia, Francesca Fremantle, Geshe Kelsang Gyatso, Charles Darwin, Henry David Thoreau, Llewellyn Vaughan-Lee, Julia Birnbaum, and Louis Fox.

With the aid of teachers of union, fast-innovating and -evolving fields such as public health and information technology may transform modernity in time to enable human survival so that the body of life will continue in the making. May human-evolved ideas and methods—theological, practical, philosophical, and scientific—enable medicine to emerge into a life-positive practice that smooths habitat restoration and integration. For my part in this opportunity I thank Hippocrates, Galen, Avicenna, Maimonides, Vesalius, and the doctors of the Scottish Enlightenment.

Last and not least, I am grateful to the Southern Oregon team that made this book beautiful. The appearance is due to the professional competence and creativity of cover artist Bruce Bayard and book designer Chris Molé. The readability is due mainly to coach Chansonette Buck and editors Deidre Krupp, Deborah Mokma, and Ann DiSalvo.

Such writing ability as I am developing, I owe first to my father, who taught me reading and writing at a young age. I am also grateful to editor friends Eva Silverfine and Stephanie Holt for their talent and skill in verbal expression, to writing teachers Andrea Goldsmith of the Victorian Writer's Centre and Wendy Call of Hugo House. They kindly put up with an unusual and neurotoxic student, trusting that their wisdom would not go to waste.

Thank you also to my book development and beta readers, especially: Jan Agosti, Anna Barón, Jessica Bondy, Cynthia Bradley, Julie Clayton, Stephanie Holt, Christopher Howell, Joel Mason, Sara Myers Wade, Berta Nicol-Blades, and Dana Smaller. Special thanks to Jan, Anna, Julie, and Stephanie for their kindness in dark times.

About the Author

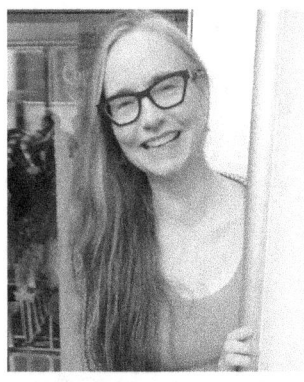

Beth Alderman, MD, MPH earned her AB and MD degrees from the University of Chicago and her MPH from the University of Washington. After Board Certification in Preventive Medicine and Public Health, she took a faculty position in the University of Colorado Medical School Department of Preventive Medicine, Biometrics, and Medical Informatics, where she did population-based epidemiological studies of adverse reproductive outcomes and methodological studies in clinical epidemiology. In her next faculty position at the University of Washington School of Public Health, she focused on risk factors for birth defects.

In 1996, she fell ill with the mysterious new plague and was given the provisional diagnosis "chronic fatigue syndrome". She has spent her time since studying her own case and pondering the reasons that her beloved profession failed her so completely. Fortunately, she discovered her cure, which may be of use to others suffering from one or more of the emerging epidemics affecting humans, their habitats, and life on earth.

For more about and from the author, see the following websites:

BethAldermanMD.com	*Free Information for all readers*
DoctorsOfLife.com	*For care and cure of all lives as one*
LivingFutureBooks.com	*Publishing Website*
LivingFutureCourses.com	*Educational Website with Free and advanced Courses*

Look for author's books on Amazon.com

Other Books by
Beth Alderman

Medical Phenomenology:
Chronic Ambient Poisoning

ISBN: 978-1-7332849-2-9

One day in December of 1996, the author (a physician, medical detective, and academic epidemiologist) developed disabling brain fog following on a decade-long descent into a painful, pervasive, and unprecedented chronic illness. Having done population-based studies to research the causes of birth defects, and having thus encountered the limitations of modern methods, she had inadvertently prepared to investigate the causes of her illness—which was given the provisional and uninformative label of "chronic fatigue."

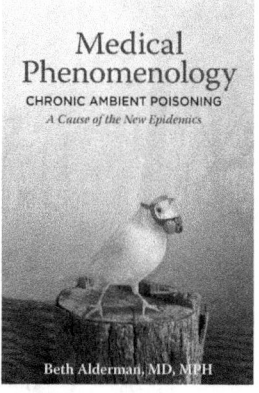

The author began a delineation of the natural history of her condition using the methods of: doctors Hippocrates, Maimonides and Oliver Sacks; the "radical empiricism" used by Dr. William James; and the phenomenology introduced by Teilhard de Chardin and Merleau-Ponty. After a fifteen-year search, she found a doctor of integrative medicine whose elimination diet relieved her brain fog, which enabled her to complete a self-study and to construct an actionable new diagnosis: chronic ambient poisoning. Unseen by doctors and obscured by medical dogma and a myriad of false diagnoses, chronic ambient poisoning defies late modern, fragmented, accuracy-challenged medical research methods and delivery systems. It also reveals that human-caused habitat injuries that afflict birds, bees, and other species are affecting humans while driving evolved life toward extinction in the way of an asteroid strike. To ignore this diagnosis is to ignore the dangers to all lives posed by maladaptive modern lifeways.

The Evolve Fertility Series

BOOK 1
Melissa's Match: *Great Society*
ISBN: 978-1-7321110-1-1

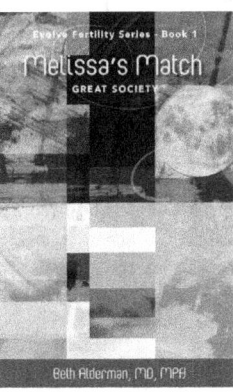

It's the early 1970s. Melissa and her friends begin their first year of college in the inner city of Chicago at a time when post-assassination riots, Great Society scholarship programs, and veterans returning from Vietnam create a sometimes explosive confluence of urban and rural, rich and poor, white and black, educated and uneducated. Coming of age in a violent, unjust, and yet hopeful time, they struggle to reconcile their hopes and opportunities with the shadows of war and the destructive clashes of senescing and emerging systems of care and cure of life on earth.

BOOK 2
Connie's Conception: *Awareness of Peril*
ISBN: 978-1-7321110-0-4

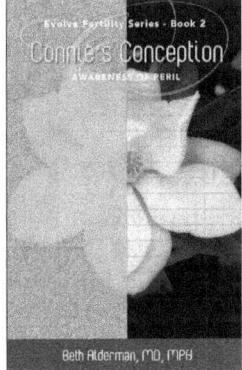

It's the late 1980s, and Connie Martin, a doctor working for the Epidemiology Intelligence Service of the CDC, is called to Colorado to investigate an alarming outbreak of birth defects. Born illegitimate in the San Luis Valley as Consuela Martín, a name known only to close friends and to her beloved gamer and programmer husband, she arrives as an unknown. Joined by environmental activists who suspect the state's Superfund sites and by doctors and parents who fear for its children, Connie attempts to discover the link between habitat destruction and damage to innocents.

BOOK 3
Melissa's Malady: *End of Modernity*
ISBN: 978-1-7321110-2-8

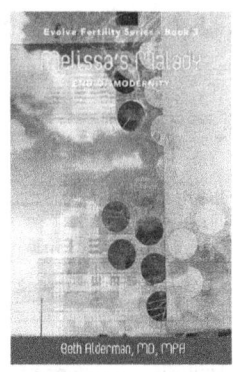

IIt is almost the year of the millennium, and Melissa meets her college friends Sarah and Doug and her first and only true love John for a reunion in Hyde Park. All four are in the midst of their careers. All struggle with the compromises that have marred their happiness. All wish to change the world, each in a different way. Sarah has left her government job for a new life as a yoga teacher. Doug is helping to birth a new value-based economy. John is a successful academic doctor. Melissa is ailing. They unite to turn John's success as a researcher to the cure of Melissa's mysterious chronic illness. What they find will change their lives and their imperiled world.

BOOK 4
Colette's Creativity: *Sacred and Profane*
ISBN: 978-1-7321110-3-5

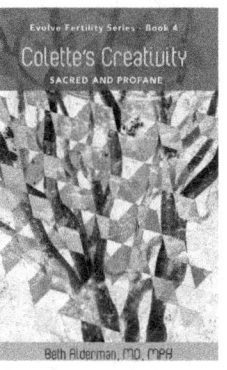

Colette, Melissa's childhood friend, abandons her marriage and home in Maine and flies to Melbourne. There she is taken in by her friend Reggie, who seems to know the secret of joy. Colette joins in the lives of striking individuals who lead her to view sexuality as a manifestation of the sacred. As she leaves behind the wounds caused by profane sexuality, she and her new friends clash with members of Reggie's family who force them to flee and to begin again.

BOOK 5
Colette's Community: *Thirds*
ISBN: 978-1-7321110-4-2

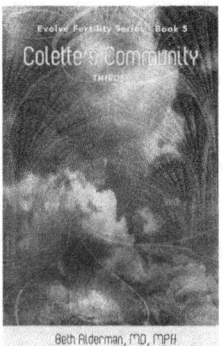

Soon after Colette and her friends find a new home, an old boyfriend of Melissa's who is sojourning in Australia calls and expresses his desire to visit. Colette plans to use the visit as a chance to develop a job for herself; he plans to check up on Colette for Melissa. As they get to know each other, they see that despite differences in religion, origin, and experience, they are on very similar spiritual paths. When it is time for Randall to go home, Colette joins him in Chicago. When he becomes caught up in his old life, however, she returns to Australia to pursue her dream of giving birth to a sacred community.

Chronic Illness Owner's Manuals
Regenerate Your Life: Chronic Illness as a Springboard for Creating Your Best Life

ISBN: 978-1-7321110-8-0 (VOL. 1)

ISBN: 978-1-7321110-9-7 (VOL. 2)

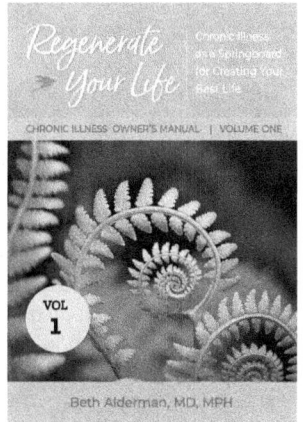

The *Chronic Illness Owner's Manual* series is for patients with chronic illness, and for the people who care for them. Suitable for individual or small group use, it offers a comprehensive, systematic, step-by-step approach to engaging modern medical systems, and to healing from the inside out.

The books comprise anecdotes, exercises, and quotes that address recovery through seven aspects of the body: awareness, understanding, perceptions, sensations, energy, flesh, and interbeing. The frames, constructs, patterns, and processes employed by the series are drawn from traditions of medicine, field biology, theology, and psychology from around the globe. Their synthesis offers an emerging, sustainable, eco-centric, eco-contextual, and customizable approach to creating a new and better life that regenerates your unique meaning, purpose, and vision of abundant life. The *Chronic Illness Owner's Manual* series complements care and cure courses available online at www. LivingFutureCourses.com.

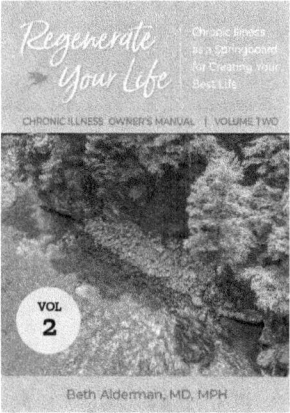

The Evolve Restoration Series
Sequel to the Evolve Fertility Series

BOOK 1
Pilgrim Minds: *After the War on Life*
ISBN: 978-1-7321110-5-9

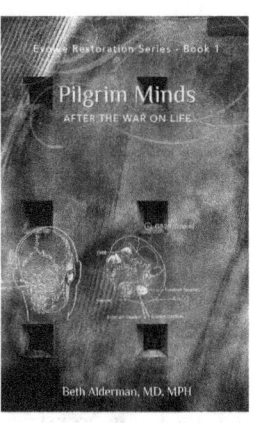

Melissa's deathbed request catapults her son Aaron on a journey from her family's Mississippian clinic to the Salish Sea to claim a mysterious legacy. Meeting his niece Rafa en route, he continues overland with her, and uncle and niece come to know and depend on each other. On arriving at the Saltspring Island Research Center (SIRC), Sarah, now the keeper of the center's narratives, confesses that Aaron's legacy is a task: to apply his mother's philosophy to SIRC's lifeways in order to revitalize it.

While he had been immersed in his mother's medical philosophy, SIRC had used many of her ideas to found a fertility school. SIRC's encroaching apathy persuaded Sarah that they missed one or more essential lifeways, and hopes that Aaron may be able to pinpoint and provide them. Taken by surprise, but ready to step up, Aaron immerses himself in the community, and Rafa undergoes SIRC's initiation process. Uncle and niece come to love Cascadia and to relish local, burgeoning patterns of innovation. Both choose to stay at SIRC, an agentic community that is doing much to restore evolution and its living future.

BOOK 2
Aaron's Legacy: *The Body of Life*
ISBN: 978-1-7321110-6-6

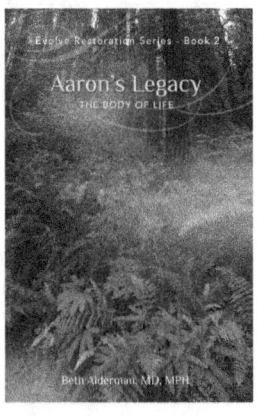

Having come to know the community, Aaron receives his legacy as a series of enactments of SIRC's history. The surviving members of his mother's old friendship group—Sarah, Doug, and John—join the audience and performers in processing and adapting their shared narrative. In the intervals between enactments, Rafa undergoes initiation while Aaron explores the composer, an instrument that enables a player to evoke memories with images and to express the player's responses as sound scapes. As Aaron shares his with Rafa, Sarah and others, John shares memories of Melissa, and seems to receive a new message from her.

As the community adapts to changes in its meaning and purpose, Rafa and Aaron each finds a first consort and draws inspiration from local knowledge keepers and change agents residing at SIRC, the nearby Monastery of Origins and Endings, or in Victoria or Vancouver. Aaron's health, damaged by his travel through a poison barren, deteriorates. With his death, his consort Parvati shares their legacy in the form of patterns of action that may remove roadblocks to continuous adaptation and renewal.

BOOK 3
The Kindred's Rebirth: *Rough Seas and Far Lands*

ISBN: 978-1-7332849-3-6

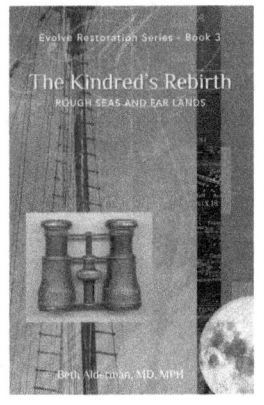

A decade later in Australia, Parvati and Björn give up on effecting meaningful restoration there. Dirk, while on his annual circuit of the north, arrives in Jokkmokk for the annual Sámi gathering to learn that SIRC is in crisis. Rafa, who is crossing the South Pacific on her two year global clinic circuit, hears strange news: the Fertility School, which was winding down, closed without notice. She realizes that her work, too, is drawing to a close as her clinics adapt to localism and begin to diverge.

All three travelers feel a strong homing urge and hatch a plan to converge in Scandinavia with the remnant of the SIRC community. En route, Parvati adopts a grandchild, Jacki, who helps Björn to recover from a disorder of interbeing. Many new consort pairs join the kindred and revive it by helping to form a next community, SIRC-Umea, and to organize and maintain residential restoration communities in the Baltic and North Sea bioregions, and to recover from the painful loss of the original community.

BOOK 4
Jacki's Vision: *The Green Line*
ISBN: 978-1-7332849-4-3

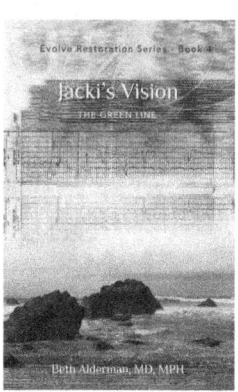

When Jacki turns sixteen, she begins her transition to adulthood by venturing into larger worlds of knowledge and adaptation to gain skills. During her first clinic circuit in the Baltic, she finds that her coming of age is coinciding with her kindred's restiveness. As she embraces and contemplates her future, a vision takes hold of her. She proposes a Green Line restoration project in Tasmania to reconcile a time debt created by the Black Line genocide, and to prepare her for organizing bioregional restoration projects. Her kindred and their networks embrace the project, expand it, and multiply its potential effects.

As the Green Line Corps prepares to depart en masse for Tasmania, Jacki meets a young stranger, Mirek, whose experience of the world—whose very umwelt—contrasts with her own. Later, in Tasmania, she gains a consort, Izaak, and a sister friend, Lally, both of whom winnow her possible futures. Together, the many thousands of Green Line participants develop a restoration ethos and synchronize living processes for restoring habitats—with their restorers. Jacki and her new peers are among the first to return to the original SIRC campus, near which many former kindred members have settled, and to which many others are about to return.

BOOK 5
Mel's Motherhood: *A Place in the Living World*
ISBN: 978-1-7332849-5-0

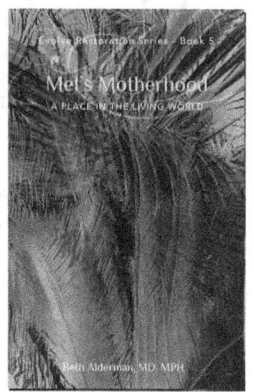

Mel and JJ—children of the Three Mammas—await the advance boat from Tasmania at the Cascadian Monastery of Origins and Endings. Mel, who is pregnant, and JJ, who fared poorly while he was away, finished their initiation projects and are keen to see Jacki and to meet the new kindred members. In the course of a joyful reunion, Mel and JJ learn that Jacki and Lally are also pregnant.

As this next generation of adults chooses ways to express fertility and defines new vocations, the reconstituting kindred celebrates new human lives, integrates with local communities, and processes hitherto hidden threads of SIRC's history with the aid of DNA fathers who participate. The complex, complementary communities adapt to continuous learning via phenomenology, and to continuous adaptation of systems for care and cure of evolved life.

Meaningful Retirement: *Become a Life Care Provider*

ISBN: 978-1-7332849-0-5

Meaningful Retirement is a self-guided monthly course in four seasons that can aid people like you who are exiting modern employment or withdrawing from the modern death economy. In it you will find a toolbox for transition to a vocation of life care, and thus begin to mature into a wise elder able to lead and mentor those who follow you. These seasons include:

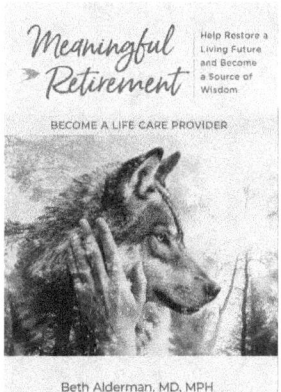

Beth Alderman, MD, MPH

- **A Summer Breather**
- **A Fall for Reflection**
- **A Winter to Reclaim Your Personal Narrative**
- **A Spring for Revolutionizing Your Lifetime Learning**

As you transition to the role of provider of life care, you may choose to co-found emotionally and spiritually astute communities where you can mentor your juniors, who face the imminent and daunting task of passing through wrenching psycho-social change while arresting and reversing the accelerating human-caused Sixth Extinction. That threat to evolved life represents a unique crucible for transforming modern lifeways into ones that enable humans to choose and to restore life. Re-visioning and co-creating processes of care and cure that restore all lives as one will prepare your species to restore the planet's living lungs, its water circulation, its living shade, and its evolved resilience to unexpected planetary catastrophes. By viewing life in time though an eco-centric and eco-contextualized lens that scales from your lifetime to evolutionary time, you can begin to see your world through new eyes that reveal your place in the big picture of life on earth.

Direct learning, that is, phenomenology, is essential for restoration of a living future. This method has changed with every epoch since ancient natural historians began to attempt to create views, frames, and constructs in an attempt to grasp evolving generative systems. The present moment of peril can be taken as an impetus and inspiration to engage with an exciting process of learning and problem solving that some call the living paradigm. This paradigm, which is still incubating in fields as diverse as architecture and design, agriculture, archaeology, restoration, and theology, is ripe for grass roots syncreses across outdated fields of knowledge. When you learn to cooperate with the last hundreds of millions of years of evolution while pursuing space age ways of averting asteroid collision, you will be prepared to lead your species toward sustainability and to make room for rapid human adaptation that restores evolution. Welcome to the One Life..